Molecular Pathology

Editor

MARTIN H. BLUTH

CLINICS IN LABORATORY MEDICINE

www.labmed.theclinics.com

Editorial Board
MATTHEW R. PINCUS
ALEXANDER J. MCADAM
KENT LEWANDROWSKI
ELLINOR PEERSCHKE

December 2013 • Volume 33 • Number 4

ELSEVIER

1600 John F. Kennedy Boulevard • Suite 1800 • Philadelphia, Pennsylvania, 19103-2899

http://www.theclinics.com

CLINICS IN LABORATORY MEDICINE Volume 33, Number 4
December 2013 ISSN 0272-2712, ISBN-13: 978-0-323-26104-3

Editor: Patrick Manley
Developmental Editor: Donald Mumford

Reprints. For copies of 100 or more, of articles in this publication, please contact the Commercial Reprints Department, Elsevier Inc., 360 Park Avenue South, New York, New York 10010-1710. Tel. 212-633-3874, Fax: 212-633-3820, E-mail: reprints@elsevier.com.

Clinics in Laboratory Medicine (ISSN 0272-2712) is published quarterly by Elsevier Inc., 360 Park Avenue South, New York, NY 10010-1710. Months of issue are March, June, September, and December. Business and Editorial offices: 1600 John F. Kennedy Blvd., Suite 1800, Philadelphia, PA 19103-2899. Periodicals postage paid at NewYork, NY and additional mailing offices. Subscription prices are $250.00 per year (US individuals), $419.00 per year (US institutions), $135.00 per year (US students), $305.00 per year (Canadian individuals), $510.00 per year (Canadian institutions), $185.00 per year (Canadian students), $390.00 per year (foreign individuals), $510.00 per year (foreign institutions), $185.00 (foreign students). Foreign air speed delivery is included in all Clinics subscription prices. All prices are subject to change without notice. POSTMASTER: Send address changes to *Clinics in Laboratory Medicine*, Elsevier Health Sciences Division, Subscription Customer Service, 3251 Riverport Lane, Maryland Heights, MO 63043. **Customer Service: 1-800-654-2452 (US). From outside of the US and Canada, call 1-314-447-8871. Fax: 1-314-447-8029. E-mail: journalscustomerservice-usa@elsevier.com (for print support) or journalsonlinesupport-usa@elsevier.com (for online support).**

Clinics in Laboratory Medicine is covered in *EMBASE/Exerpta Medica, MEDLINE/PubMed (Index Medicus), Cinahl, Current Contents/Clinical Medicine, BIOSIS and ISI/BIOMED.*

Printed and bound by CPI Group (UK) Ltd, Croydon, CR0 4YY

Transferred to digital print 2013

Contributors

EDITOR

MARTIN H. BLUTH, MD, PhD
Professor of Pathology, Karmanos Cancer Institute, Detroit Medical Center, Wayne State University School of Medicine, Detroit, Michigan

AUTHORS

QURATULAIN AHMED, MD
Fellow, Department of Pathology, Wayne State University, Detroit, Michigan

SHADAN ALI, MS
Department of Oncology, Karmanos Cancer Institute, Wayne State University School of Medicine, Detroit, Michigan

ROUBA ALI-FEHMI, MD
Professor, Department of Pathology, Wayne State University, Detroit, Michigan

BARAA ALOSH, MD
Research Associate, Department of Pathology, Wayne State University, Detroit, Michigan

SUDESHNA BANDYOPADHYAY, MD
Assistant Professor, Department of Pathology, Wayne State University, Detroit, Michigan

AMARPREET BHALLA, MBBS, MD
Senior Resident, (PGY-3), Pathology Department, Harper University Hospital, Detroit Medical Center, Wayne State University School of Medicine, Detroit, Michigan

MARK J. BLUTH, PhD
Senior Scientist, Genome Dynamics International, Uniondale, New York

MARTIN H. BLUTH, MD, PhD
Professor of Pathology, Karmanos Cancer Institute, Detroit Medical Center, Wayne State University School of Medicine, Detroit, Michigan

ROBERTSON D. DAVENPORT, MD
Department of Pathology, University of Michigan Health System, Ann Arbor, Michigan

MATTHEW B. ELKINS, MD, PhD
Department of Pathology, Upstate Medical University, Syracuse, New York

MARILYNN RANSOM FAIRFAX, MD, PhD
Associate Professor of Pathology, Wayne State University School of Medicine; Staff Pathologist, Microbiology Division, Detroit Medical Center University Laboratories, Detroit, Michigan

ALI M. GABALI, MD, PhD
Department of Pathology, Karmanos Cancer Institute, Detroit Medical Center, Wayne State University, Detroit, Michigan

TAREK JAZAERLY, MD
Department of Pathology, Karmanos Cancer Institute, Detroit Medical Center, Wayne State University, Detroit, Michigan

DEJUAN KONG, PhD
Department of Pathology, Karmanos Cancer Institute, Wayne State University School of Medicine, Detroit, Michigan

BARBARA A. O'MALLEY, MD
Department of Pathology, Detroit Medical Center, Wayne State University, Detroit, Michigan

PHILIP A. PHILIP, MD, PhD
Department of Oncology, Karmanos Cancer Institute, Wayne State University School of Medicine, Detroit, Michigan

RADHAKRISHNAN RAMCHANDREN, MD
Department of Hematology/Oncology, Karmanos Cancer Institute, Detroit Medical Center, Wayne State University, Detroit, Michigan

HOSSEIN SALIMNIA, PhD
Associate Professor of Pathology, Wayne State University School of Medicine; Technical Chief, Microbiology Division, Detroit Medical Center University Laboratories, Detroit, Michigan

FAZLUL H. SARKAR, PhD
Departments of Pathology and Oncology, Karmanos Cancer Institute, Wayne State University School of Medicine, Detroit, Michigan

SEEMA SETHI, MD
Department of Pathology, Karmanos Cancer Institute, Wayne State University School of Medicine, Detroit, Michigan

VINOD B. SHIDHAM, MD, FRCPath, FIAC
Vice Chair, Anatomical Pathology; Professor and Director of Cytopathology, Department of Pathology, Karmanos Cancer Center, Detroit Medical Center, Wayne State University School of Medicine, Detroit, Michigan

ANDREW DAVID THOMPSON, MD, PhD, FCAP
Department of Pathology, DMC Harper University Hospital, Wayne State University School of Medicine; Barbara Ann Karmanos Cancer Institute, Detroit, Michigan

MICHAEL WEINDEL, MD
Assistant Professor, Department of Pathology, Karmanos Cancer Center, Detroit Medical Center, Wayne State University School of Medicine, Detroit, Michigan

MUHAMMAD ZULFIQAR, MD
Fellow, Cytopathology, (PGY-5), Pathology Department, Detroit Medical Center, Wayne State University School of Medicine, Detroit, Michigan; Hematopathology Fellow, Department of Pathology and Laboratory Medicine, Indiana University School of Medicine, Indianapolis, Indiana

Contents

Molecular pathology is affecting and influencing the entire clinical laboratory. Furthermore, the union of pathology and molecular medicine continues
to mature into an amalgam that will both define and serve the emerging field
of personalized medicine. Advances in the understanding of pathobiology,
high throughput automation, cost containment, and refined methodology
will avail greater diagnostic and prognostic prowess and provide more efficient and appropriate therapeutic selection as well guide effective patient
monitoring with respect to disease responses.

Molecular pathology techniques have matured considerably over the
last decade. New technologies have provided increased sensitivity for
improved diagnostic capacity. Furthermore, novel methodologies have
matured to interrogate nucleic acid and protein signatures effectively to
aid in elucidating the pathophysiology of disease in addition to diagnosis,
prognosis, and therapeutic monitoring for patient management. Here general molecular techniques used in the molecular pathology laboratory as
they are used for clinical applications are described.

MicroRNAs are small endogenous noncoding RNAs that are critical regu-
lators of several physiologic and pathologic processes including cancers.
Variations in the level of microRNA expression have been linked with the
development, progression, and spread of cancer to distant organs. These
tiny molecules may play a role in accurate and early diagnosis, and also as
prognostic determinants. Modulating their activity provides opportunities
for developing and designing novel cancer therapeutics. Recent studies
indicate their detection in a wide variety of human biologic specimens
including blood, serum, fine-needle aspirates, and tissues, making them
clinically useful biomarkers of disease for early detection, prognosis, and
for designing personalized therapies.

Molecular testing has a large and increasing role in the diagnosis of infectious diseases. It has evolved significantly since the first probe tests were

FDA approved in the early 1990s. This article highlights the uses of molecular techniques in diagnostic microbiology, including "older," as well as innovative, probe techniques, qualitative and quantitative RT-PCR, highly multiplexed PCR panels, some of which use sealed microfluidic test cartridges, MALDI TOF, and nuclear magnetic resonance. Tests are grouped together by technique and target. Tests with similar roles for similar analytes are compared with respect to benefits, drawbacks, and possible problems.

This article provides an overview of the application of molecular diagnostic methods to red cell and platelet compatibility testing. The advantages and limitations of molecular methods are evaluated compared with traditional serologic methods. The molecular bases of clinically significant red cell and platelet antigens are presented. Current recommendations for reporting molecular assay results and distinctions between genotype and phenotype are discussed.

Cytogenetic abnormalities are considered to be common events in hematologic malignancies. These abnormalities generally consist of structural chromosomal abnormalities or gene mutations, which often are integral to the pathogenesis and subsequent evolution of an individual malignancy. Improvements made in identifying and interpreting these molecular alterations have resulted in advances in the diagnosis, prognosis, monitoring, and therapy for cancer. As a consequence of the increasingly important role of molecular testing in hematologic malignancy management, this article presents an update on the importance and use of molecular tests, detailing the advantages and disadvantages of each test when applicable.

Molecular pathogenesis and classification of colorectal carcinoma are based on the adenoma-carcinoma sequence in the Vogelstein model, serrated polyp pathway, and microsatellite instability. The genetic basis for hereditary nonpolyposis colorectal cancer is based on detection of genetic mutations. Genetic testing for Lynch syndrome includes microsatellite instability, methylator phenotyping, BRAF mutation, and molecular testing. Molecular makers include quantitative multigene reverse transcriptase–polymerase chain reaction assay and KRAS and BRAF mutation analysis. Potential biomarkers include one-step nucleic acid amplification and epigenetic inactivation of endothelin 2 and endothelin 3 in colon cancer. Molecular screening approaches in colorectal cancer using stool DNA are under investigation.

treatments. This article discusses how these technologies are altering the ways in which cutaneous melanocytic neoplasms are diagnosed and treated.

The most significant contribution of molecular subtyping of breast carcinomas has been the identification of estrogen-positive and estrogen-negative tumor subtypes, which are 2 distinct entities with differing prognoses and requiring different therapy. Molecular and genetic analyses can provide prognostic information; however, a thorough histopathologic evaluation with an evaluation of predictive biomarkers will provide similar information. Knowledge of genetic alterations in these tumors will help identify novel therapeutic targets, which might have an impact on prognosis. Understanding the progression pathways involved in the transition of in situ carcinoma to invasive carcinoma might lead to efficient risk stratification in these patients.

This article reviews the molecular features and pathogenesis of gynecologic malignancies. Understanding the molecular basis of endometrial carcinoma helps to provide an explanation for the prognosis of these tumors and opens up avenues for research into novel therapies that may prove beneficial.

CLINICS IN LABORATORY MEDICINE

FORTHCOMING ISSUES

March 2014
Cardiac Markers
Kent Lewandrowski, MD, *Editor*

June 2014
Respiratory Infections
Michael Loeffelholz, PhD, D(ABMM),
Editor

September 2014
Anticoagulants
Jerrold H. Levy, MD, FAHA, FCCM, and
Ingrid Pabinger-Fasching, MD, *Editors*

RECENT ISSUES

September 2013
**Automation and Emerging Technology in
Clinical Microbiology**
Carey-Ann D. Burnham, PhD, D(ABMM),
F(CCM), *Editor*

June 2013
**Diabetes, Hematology/Coagulation in
Pregnancy**
Winston A. Campbell, MD, *Editor*

March 2013
**Quality Control in the Age of Risk
Management**
James O. Westgard, PhD, FACB and
Sten Westgard, MS, *Editors*

Preface

Molecular Pathology in the Modern Era: Revisiting Jacob's Spotted Sheep

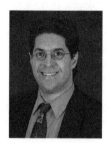

Martin H. Bluth, MD, PhD
Editor

The Bible recounts the tumultuous story of the patriarch Jacob during his sojourn in the House of Laban in his quest to betroth the matriarch Rachel. Despite Laban's continuous trickery, deception, and debauchery in an effort to prohibit Jacob from claiming his due, whether in his marriage to Rachel or his earning of agreed upon wages, Jacob somewhat successfully prevails. Jacob, being attuned to Laban's malfeasance, proposes an odd request for wages. A rather obscure passage states the following: "Let me go through all your flocks today and remove from them every speckled or spotted sheep, every dark colored lamb and every spotted or speckled goat. They will be my wages."[1] The Materials and Methods section of the classic text continues, "Jacob, however, took fresh-cut branches from poplar, almond and plane trees and made white stripes on them by peeling the bark and exposing the white inner wood of the branches. Then he placed the peeled branches in all the watering troughs, so that they would be directly in front of the flocks when they came to drink. When the flocks were in heat and came to drink, they mated in front of the branches."[1] Finally, the Results section verifies that the experiment proves successful, "And they bore young that were streaked or speckled or spotted,"[1] where Jacob amasses the wealth that is due him.

Although many commentaries postulate this episode as an intended exercise using classical genetics, selective breeding, physiology, and epigenetics,[2,3] it may be equally suggestive as a model of modern day molecular medicine in animals[4] as well as in humans. Indeed, molecular medicine with respect to heredity probabilities, polymorphisms, recombination genetics, pharmacogenomics, pharmacogenetics, and the like in malignancy and other disease spaces has gained considerable popularity over the last decade with the current culmination of personalized medicine.[5,6] Whereas years ago one would subscribe to the mantra "one gene one protein" hypothesis,

Clin Lab Med 33 (2013) xi–xiii
http://dx.doi.org/10.1016/j.cll.2013.09.003
0272-2712/13/$ – see front matter © 2013 Published by Elsevier Inc.

today's medical marketplace is seeing a paradigm shift in assessing multiplex interplays of factors that demonstrate pathway effects, which are taken into account in disease diagnosis, prognosis, therapeutic intervention, and patient management strategies.[7]

Molecular pathology, the discipline within pathology that focuses on the study and diagnosis of disease through the examination of molecules within organs, tissues, or bodily fluids,[8] has evolved into the gatekeeper of molecular methodology with respect to its design, application, sensitivity, specificity, predictive value, interfering factors, and limitations to various disease spectra. The modern day pathologist is no longer limited to the microscope, paying homage to Leeuwenhoek's lens craftsmanship. Rather, the molecular pathologist is an all encompassing tour de force who is versed in molecular, cellular, and architectural aspects of tissue with respect to disease as well as its relationship to the multifactorial nature of its clinical presentation, variation, and polymorphism, which can often present confounding issues pertaining to diagnostic prowess.

The diagnostic methodological armamentarium has expanded considerably to include interrogation of nucleic acid—encompassing polymerase chain reaction (PCR) and its permutations (ie, real-time PCR), FISH, SNPs, and miRNA, among others—as well as protein assessment (ie, ELISA, Western Blot, IHC). Furthermore, the "omics" explosion, presenting a unique manner of high throughput technologies, will also further expound on disease from a biological systems approach.[9] In addition, cellular and tissue microarrays[10,11] hold additional promise for biomarker discovery, development, maturation, and application to various diseases.

To this end, the molecular pathologist may be likened to a modern day "molecular shepherd," who will facilitate the evolution of the personalized medicine era and translate such into cogent, meaningful laboratory data toward the application to disease diagnosis, prognosis, and patient management for the betterment of mankind.

Martin H. Bluth, MD, PhD
Professor of Pathology
Karmanos Cancer Institute
Detroit Medical Center
Wayne State University School of Medicine
8203 Scott Hall
540 E. Canfield
Detroit, MI 48201, USA

E-mail address:
mbluth@med.wayne.edu

REFERENCES

1. Genesis 30:32–43.
2. Available at: http://www.volconvo.com/forums/religion-spirituality/27347-science-jacobs-spotted-sheep.html.
3. Available at: http://jbq.jewishbible.org/assets/Uploads/364/364_sheep.pdf.
4. Hall IM, Quinlan AR. Detection and interpretation of genomic structural variation in mammals. Methods Mol Biol 2012;838:225–48.
5. Mendelsohn J. Personalizing oncology: perspectives and prospects. J Clin Oncol 2013;31:1904–11.
6. Johnson JA, Cavallari LH. Pharmacogenetics and cardiovascular disease—implications for personalized medicine. Pharmacol Rev 2013;65:987–1009.

7. Starčević JN, Petrovič D. Carotid intima media-thickness and genes involved in lipid metabolism in diabetic patients using statins—a pathway toward personalized medicine. Cardiovasc Hematol Agents Med Chem 2013;11:3–8.
8. Available at: http://en.wikipedia.org/wiki/Molecular_pathology.
9. Chen R, Snyder M. Promise of personalized omics to precision medicine. Wiley Interdiscip Rev Syst Biol Med 2013;5:73–82.
10. Papp K, Szittner Z, Prechl J. Life on a microarray: assessing live cell functions in a microarray format. Cell Mol Life Sci 2012;69:2717–25.
11. Franco R, Caraglia M, Facchini G, et al. The role of tissue microarray in the era of target-based agents. Expert Rev Anticancer Ther 2011;11:859–69.

Introduction: The Impact of Molecular Pathology on the Practice of Pathology

Martin H. Bluth, MD, PhD

KEYWORD

- Molecular pathology • Methods • Genomics • High throughput • Quality
- Polymorphisms

KEY POINTS

- The Human Genome Project has paved the way for molecular pathology to profoundly influence general pathology practice and the understanding of pathobiology.
- Molecular pathology techniques have provided medicine with accurate, sensitive, and rapid opportunities to diagnose and prognosticate disease in an unprecedented manner.
- Application of molecular pathology to high-throughput automation is providing the ability for multiplex analysis and personalized medicine for individual patients.
- Detection of abnormal genes and differences in patterns of gene expression can influence disease diagnosis and guide specific therapy.

The success of the Human Genome Project[1] has expanded the field of molecular biology in an exponential manner. It has facilitated the identification of numerous novel genes of unknown function whose functions can now be determined and whose expressions can be monitored in different disease states. Whereas the discipline of pathology often refers to the rubric of the study of disease in general, molecular pathology refers to the analysis of nucleic acids and proteins to diagnose disease, predict the occurrence of disease, and predict the prognosis of diagnosed disease and guide therapy.

Furthermore, recent advances in molecular pathology have positively affected the practice of medicine, especially diagnostic medicine. These changes result from abilities to clone disease-causing genes and the proteins that they encode and to detect the presence of these genes and proteins in the serum and other body fluids and tissues of patients, even though they may be present in minute quantities. This detection has been made possible by a veritable explosion of new, highly sensitive techniques involving amplification methods, such as polymerase chain reaction, branched DNA,

Karmanos Cancer Institute, Detroit Medical Center, Wayne State University School of Medicine, 8203 Scott Hall, 540 East Canfield, Detroit, MI 48201, USA
E-mail address: mbluth@med.wayne.edu

Clin Lab Med 33 (2013) 749–751
http://dx.doi.org/10.1016/j.cll.2013.09.002   labmed.theclinics.com
0272-2712/13/$ – see front matter © 2013 Elsevier Inc. All rights reserved.

fluorescence in situ hybridization, and mass spectroscopy, among others. The ability to streamline testing in a high-throughput manner, many of which have been automated, enables a single patient sample to be analyzed for multiple genes or proteins.

Molecular pathology has afforded physicians the ability to drill down into interrogating disease states for causes related to chromosomal abnormalities, point mutations, polymorphisms, and the like, which can provide a personalized medicine approach to diagnose a wide spectrum of diseases. To this end, genes that encode drug-metabolizing enzymes, both activating and inactivating, and genes that encode ligands and receptors may show polymorphisms that either decrease or increase the therapeutic effectiveness or toxicity of drugs already in clinical use, thus accounting for some idiosyncratic responses previously not understood or predictable. As such, there have been major advances in testing patients for genetic expression of selective enzyme isoforms, allowing prediction of which drugs would be the most effective ones.

As more polymorphisms are identified and correlated with individual patients' response to treatment, pathologists will be called on increasingly to profile common polymorphisms in patients who are beginning therapy for common diseases, such as coronary artery disease, congestive heart failure, diabetes, thrombosis, hypertension, cancer, and infections. Mutations in select genes, produced by mutational events associated with, for instance, carcinogens and oncogenic viruses, often result in abnormal activation or overexpression of their encoded proteins. A laboratory's definition of an individual patient's genotype/phenotype, therefore, may determine the specific drugs and doses suitable for the patient. This evolution has placed pathologists in a more definitive position to determine appropriate therapy than traditional prediction of disease behavior based on morphology of lesions or culture characteristics of infectious organisms.[2]

Cancer is a major area in which the differential expression of specific genes characterizes particular tumors. New advances in molecular pathology related to gynecology, gastroenterology, dermatology, and hematology disciplines have provided unprecedented insight into the diagnosis of and screening for several different types of tumors. Similar advances have been accomplished in the disciplines of infectious disease and transfusion medicine. Clinical laboratories will likely be called on to perform such in-depth types of analyses with increasing frequency in the near future.

A poignant example of this phenomenon is the diagnosis of leukemias and lymphomas. Morphologically and even immunophenotypically, it may prove difficult to distinguish among different types of each disease. Specific gene rearrangements and patterns of gene expression, however, now enable distinction of different types of disease in this regard. In addition, the relationships among diseases are also more sharply defined, and sometimes radically changed, by comparisons among the diseases' gene expression profiles.[3,4]

As with all laboratory methods, excellent quality-assurance programs are required to ensure that molecular pathologic results are accurate and useful. Standardized methods for performance of the most common clinical molecular pathologic tests are published by the Clinical and Laboratory Standards Institute (formerly called the National Committee for Clinical Laboratory Standards). Use of these guidelines ensures that the data generated in molecular pathology laboratories are produced by methods that are the standard of excellent practice. Furthermore, interlaboratory comparison of test performance is provided by the College of American Pathologists (www.cap.org). Applying established standards of quality assurance and using molecular pathologic techniques with a thorough understanding of their respective strengths and weaknesses, pathologists will continue to capitalize on the opportunities these techniques offer for improved patient care and the understanding of basic pathobiology.

Financial costs inherent in operations pertaining to a molecular pathology laboratory need to be considered as well. Although molecular pathology tests can often incur higher costs than conventional testing approaches, there are proponents who argue that molecular testing may actually facilitate a decrease in unnecessary, less-sensitive, and less-specific tests, thereby perpetuating more targeted and appropriate therapy for patients in the long run.[5,6]

In summary, molecular diagnostic techniques provide new insights into disease that were never before possible. These techniques, however, must often be used in coordination with traditional laboratory tests. In cases of tissue pathology, the morphologic skills involved in histopathology and cytopathology must be used to ensure that appropriate cells and tissues are analyzed molecularly. Otherwise, analysis of other than targeted cells/tissues, despite high-quality technical methods interpreted with skill and experience, can lead to erroneous, sometimes dangerously misleading, results. In concert with classical pathology algorithms, molecular pathology affords unprecedented potential for refined, highly sensitive, rapid, and patient-specific characterization of disease. To this end, molecular pathologists are situated as proverbial diagnostic gatekeepers to ascertain and affirm that the evolution of molecular medicine is handled, processed, and interpreted appropriately for optimal patient care.

REFERENCES

1. Venter JC, Adams MD, Myers EW, et al. The sequence of the human genome. Science 2001;291:1304–51.
2. Tozzi V. Pharmacogenetics of antiretrovirals. Antiviral Res 2010;85:190–200.
3. Bacher U, Kohlmann A, Haferlach T. Current status of gene expression profiling in the diagnosis and management of acute leukaemia. Br J Haematol 2009;145: 555–68.
4. Talaulikar D, Dahlstrom JE. Staging bone marrow in diffuse large B-cell lymphoma: the role of ancillary investigations. Pathology 2009;41:214–22.
5. Ross JS. The impact of molecular diagnostic tests on patient outcomes. Clin Lab Med 1999;19:815–31.
6. Ross JS. Financial determinants of outcomes in molecular testing. Arch Pathol Lab Med 1999;123:1071–5.

Molecular Pathology Techniques

Mark J. Bluth, PhD[a],*, Martin H. Bluth, MD, PhD[b]

KEYWORDS

- Molecular pathology • Methodology • RT-PCR • FISH • RFLP • SNP
- Hybrid capture

KEY POINTS

- Polymerase chain reaction (PCR) remains the cornerstone methodology for nucleic acid amplification.
- Improvements on nucleic acid detection methodologies (ie, PCR) have increased the detection sensitivity by using fluorescent and bead array–based technologies.
- Single base-pair lesions can be detected via sequencing and related techniques to discern point mutations in disease pathogenesis.
- Novel technologies such as high-resolution melting analysis provide fast, high-throughput post-PCR analysis of genetic mutations or variance in nucleic acid sequences.
- Infectious disease can now be detected by fluorophore or chemiluminescent detection assays, such as Hybrid Capture hybridization technology, allowing for rapid diagnosis.

POLYMERASE CHAIN REACTION

Polymerase chain reaction (PCR) is a chemical reaction that facilitates the in vitro synthesis of potentially unlimited quantities of a targeted nucleic acid sequence. Basically, the reaction consists of a target DNA molecule, an excess of the forward and reverse oligonucleotide primers (typically 15–30 nucleotides long), a thermostable DNA polymerase (typically *Taq* or *Pfu*), an equimolar mixture of deoxyribonucleotide triphosphates (dATP, dCTP, dGTP, and dTTP), Mg^{2+} or Mn^{2+} (depending on the type of polymerase used), KCl, and an appropriate Tris-HCl buffer.

The reaction consists of 3 steps: denaturation, annealing, and extension, which taken together are referred to as a "cycle." To begin, the reaction mixture is heated (usually to ∼95°C) to separate the 2 strands of target DNA (denaturation) and then cooled to a temperature at which the primers will bind to the target DNA in a sequence-specific manner (annealing). Immediately after primer annealing, the DNA polymerase binds (as the temperature is raised to ∼72°C) and initiates polymerization, resulting in the extension of each primer at its 3′ end (extension). During the following cycle the primer extension products are subsequently heated to dissociate from the

a Genome Dynamics International, Uniondale, NY 11556, USA; b Karmanos Cancer Institute, Detroit Medical Center, Wayne State University School of Medicine, Detroit, Michigan
* Corresponding author.
E-mail address: mark.bluth@gendyn.us

Clin Lab Med 33 (2013) 753–772
http://dx.doi.org/10.1016/j.cll.2013.09.004   **labmed.theclinics.com**

target DNA. Each new extension product, as well as the original target, can serve as a template for subsequent rounds of primer annealing and extension. In doing so, at the end of each cycle, the PCR products are theoretically doubled.[1,2]

The whole procedure is carried out in a programmable thermocycler that precisely controls the temperature at which the steps occur, the length of time that the reaction is held at the different temperatures, and the number of cycles. Ideally, after 20 cycles of PCR, a million-fold amplification is achieved and, after 30 cycles, the replicons approach a billion-fold.

REVERSE TRANSCRIPTION PCR

As described above, PCR is suitable for the amplification of DNA targets because DNA polymerase does not recognize DNA-primed RNA templates. Reverse transcription (RT) PCR helps overcome this problem by using the enzyme reverse transcriptase to first synthesize a strand of complementary DNA (cDNA) using the RNA as a template. Because thermolabile RNA is often referred to as the message transcribed from the DNA template, this process provides a thermostable mirror image of the RNA transcript. Typically, recombinant reverse transcriptase is added to a reaction mixture identical to the one for PCR and is incubated at between 37°C and 42°C for 30 minutes during which time the first-strand cDNA synthesis occurs. Subsequently, the reaction proceeds much like a regular PCR reaction for the appropriate number of cycles at the appropriate temperatures. This method can, however, present problems in terms of both the nonspecific primer annealing and inefficient primer extension due to formation of RNA secondary structures. A secondary RNA structure is a direct consequence of the low temperature at which the reaction is carried out, due to the heat labile nature of most RTs. These problems have been largely overcome by the development of a thermostable DNA polymerase derived from *Thermus thermophilus* (ie, Taq polymerase), which, under the proper conditions, can function efficiently as both an RT and a DNA polymerase.[2]

REAL-TIME PCR

Real-time (also called "quantitative" [qPCR, qRT-PCR] or "kinetic" [kPCR, kRT-PCR]) is a closed-system assay that can be used to determine the relative quantity of gene expression as well as genotyping by detection of single-nucleotide polymorphisms (SNP).

In principle, the method works much like the PCR mentioned above; however, real-time PCR also uses an additional oligonucleotide probe. This probe is target message-specific and contains a fluorochrome at one end and a quencher molecule at the other. When unhybridized, the probe forms a hairpin structure that brings the fluorochrome in proximity with and binds the quencher, effectively muting its fluorescence. However, when hybridized, the quencher molecule is cleaved, and the bound fluorochrome is now unencumbered and can be detected by a fluorescence absorption assay. Single-nucleotide differences like SNPs can be detected in PCR products by the sequence-specific hybridization of the probe. Because it is possible to have different colored fluorochromes, the probes can be differentially labeled, allowing both alleles of an SNP to be typed in the same tube. These molecules can be used in a closed system for allelic discrimination of PCR products. Both assays can be read in real time or end-point formats, using a fluorescent thermocycler or LightCycler. This PCR-based assay can be consolidated by combining an amplification primer and the fluorescent detection component in the same molecule to enable real-time genotyping.

Once suitable oligonucleotides are designed, the genotyping of a sample is straightforward. The instrument is programed to amplify the DNA and to perform a melting curve analysis. A perfect match has a higher melting temperature than a mismatch. In this way, the LightCycler directly genotypes a sample after amplification with no additional handling. With dual-color detection, it is possible to simultaneously genotype 2 different mutations in one PCR run.[3–5]

MULTIPLEX PCR

Multiplex PCR (mpPCR) consists of multiple primer sets within a single PCR mixture to produce amplicons of differing sizes that specifically identify different DNA sequences. Primer sets are designed so that their annealing temperatures are optimized to work correctly within a single reaction. The resultant amplicons are different enough in size to form distinct bands when visualized by gel electrophoresis. By its original design, this assay is typically efficient for elucidating the presence and relative concentrations of from 2 to 20 distinct messages and is limited by the resolution capacity of electophoretic gel separation.[6]

XTAG TECHNOLOGY

xTAG technology (Luminex Corp, Austin, TX, USA) is a next-generation form of multiplexing that overcomes the resolution limits of mpPCR by combining the methods of multiplex amplification with particle-based flow cytometry. Like mpPCR, multiple reactions can be carried out in a single reaction; however, because of the added flow component, many more tests can be run and resolved at the same time.

Using a viral panel as an example, after obtaining a biologic sample, the mRNA is reverse transcribed to cDNA. The cDNA is then amplified using a panel of primers that can specifically amplify many different pathologic/pathogenic nucleic acid sequences at the same time. Each pathogen-specific primer used is tagged with a unique oligonucleotide sequence (called the tag) as well as a fluorophore. After the multiplex amplification step is completed, the reaction is mixed with microscopic beads that are internally tagged with varying amounts of fluorescent molecules at the time of production. Each different type of bead is also labeled with a unique oligonucleotide sequence that is complementary to the unique tag on the pathogen-specific primer (called the anti-tag). If both the tag and the anti-tag are present, then hybridization occurs, binding the fluorophore-labeled amplicon to its appropriate fluorophore-labeled bead. The beads are then processed and placed in a special flow-enabled luminometer equipped with 2 lasers for reading. The first of the 2 lasers identifies the bead based on its internal dye content and the second laser detects how much, if any, tagged amplicon is bound to its surface.[7]

This technology allows for the resolution of 100 or more tests from one sample at one time in one tube. It is adaptable to perform tests on nucleic acids, peptides, and proteins in a variety of sample matrixes.

STRAND DISPLACEMENT AMPLIFICATION

Strand displacement amplification method allows for rapid isothermal amplification of target nucleic acid molecules using a series of primers, DNA polymerase (exo-*Bst*), and a restriction endonuclease (*Bso*BI), to amplify a unique nucleic acid sequence exponentially.[8] *Bso*BI recognizes the nucleic acid sequence: 5′ C-(C or T)-C-G-(A or G)-G 3′. One of the primers, commonly called the "bump" primer, contains a sequence complementary to a unique target sequence, but also contains a 5′ linker with a built-in *Bso*BI restriction site.

Strand displacement amplification can be thought of as occurring in 2 segments: a target generation phase and an exponential amplification phase. In the target generation phase after the heat denaturation of the native nucleic acid, primers anneal (**Fig. 1**) and the polymerization reaction occurs in both directions in the presence of modified dCTPαS (**Fig. 2**), which results in the production of a double-stranded product with a *Bso*BI restriction site 5′ to the target sequence. Next, the *Bso*BI restriction site within the primer is digested with *Bso*BI. However, because the newly polymerized DNA strands (the strands complementary to and extended from the "bump" primer) were synthesized with dCTPαS, only one side of the *Bso*BI site is sensitive to digestion, resulting in the production of one nicked strand (**Fig. 3**). Next, the exo-*Bst* polymerase binds to the nicked strand, on the 5′ side of the nick, and polymerizes a new strand extending from the nick site, displacing the previous strand in the process. The strand is nicked again with *Bso*BI and the process repeats (**Fig. 4**). The newly displaced strand will serve as a template in following rounds of amplification. The exponential amplification phase describes the continuous repetition of this process and can produce copies in excess of a million-fold within 2 hours.[9,10]

The reaction can be performed with real-time analysis if coupled with a fluorescent probe and multiplexed via an initial purifying step in which the "bumper" primer is covalently linked to magnetic or fluorescently labeled beads.

TRANSCRIPTION-MEDIATED AMPLIFICATION

Transcription-mediated amplification (TMA) is an isothermal nucleic acid-based method that can amplify RNA or DNA targets a billion-fold in less than 1 hour (**Fig. 5**). This system is useful for detecting the presence of *Mycobacterium tuberculosis* and *Chlamydia trachomatis*.

Developed at Gen-Probe (Hologic Gen-Probe, San Diego, CA, USA), TMA technology uses 2 primers and 2 enzymes: RNA polymerase and reverse transcriptase. One primer contains a promoter sequence for RNA polymerase. In the first step of amplification, this primer hybridizes to the target rRNA at a defined site. Reverse transcriptase creates a DNA copy of the target rRNA by extension from the 3′ end of the promoter primer. The RNA in the resulting RNA:DNA duplex is degraded by the RNase activity of the reverse transcriptase. Next, a second primer binds to the DNA copy. A new strand of DNA is synthesized from the end of this primer by reverse transcriptase, creating a double-stranded DNA (dsRNA) molecule. RNA polymerase recognizes the

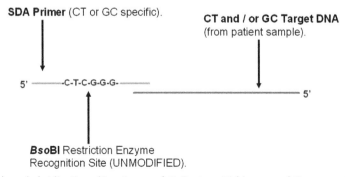

Fig. 1. Primer hybridization. (Courtesy and © Becton, Dickinson and Company. Reprinted with permission.)

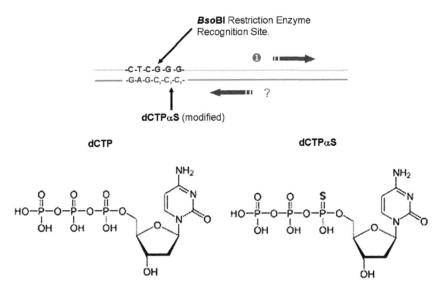

Fig. 2. Primer extension. (Courtesy and © Becton, Dickinson and Company. Reprinted with permission.)

promoter sequence in the DNA template and initiates transcription. Each of the newly synthesized RNA amplicons reenters the TMA process and serves as a template for a new round of replication. The amplicons produced in these reactions are detected by a specific gene probe via hybridization protection assay followed by a chemiluminescence detection protocol.[11,12]

DNA SEQUENCING

DNA sequencing using the enzymatic extension reaction makes use of the difference between normal deoxyribonucleotides and dideoxyribonucleotides. Deoxyribonucleotides contain a hydroxyl group at position 3 on the pentose sugar ring, allowing DNA polymerase to join it with the phosphate group of the next nucleotide. A dideoxynucleotide can be incorporated into a growing chain, but because it does not contain a hydroxyl group at position 3, no additional nucleotides can be added, effectively terminating polymerization of that chain at that point.

The reaction is the same as a standard PCR with the exception of the supplementation of a small concentration of a labeled dideoxynucleotide to the reaction mix in

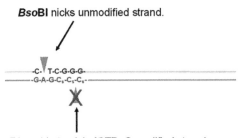

Fig. 3. Single-strand digestion. (Courtesy and © Becton, Dickinson and Company. Reprinted with permission.)

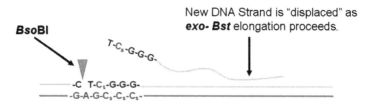

Fig. 4. Nicked-strand displacement. (Courtesy and © Becton, Dickinson and Company. Reprinted with permission.)

addition to the regular quantities of the normal deoxynucleotide triphosphates (dATP, dTTP, dCTP, and dGTP). Using dideoxythymidine triphosphate (ddTTP) as an example, the DNA to be sequenced is denatured, complementary primers anneal, and primer extension occurs as normal. However, when ddTTP is incorporated instead of dTTP, DNA polymerization on that molecule terminates. When the reaction is carried

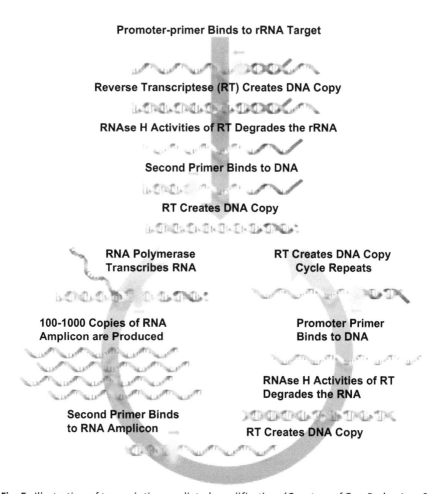

Fig. 5. Illustration of transcription mediated amplification. (*Courtesy of* Gen-Probe, Inc., San Diego, CA; with permission.)

out in the presence of the optimal concentrations of both dTTP and ddTTP, there will be molecules synthesized that stop at each of the thymidine nucleotides in the sequence. The fragments generated can then be separated out by size via gel electrophoresis and the tag on the ddNTP allows the fragment to be visualized. In the beginning, the reaction was carried out using 4 different tubes, each one containing a different ddNTP. The reaction uses radiolabeled nucleotides (ie, S^{35}), and when completed, the reactions were separated in parallel lanes of a gel (one lane per ddNTP), which was then exposed to film, yielding a staggered pattern of bands each with a one nucleotide base difference in size from the next. When the order of the bands from all 4 lanes is read in size order from bottom to top, it would correspond to the sequence of the DNA fragment that was amplified from the primer onward (**Fig. 6**).

This method is excellent for sequencing fragments up to 600 base pairs. As a result, the method could get costly for the time and reagents necessary to perform multiple reactions required to verify the sequence of longer DNA fragments. Today, however, the same reaction can be performed using ddNTPs labeled with different fluorophores in one tube, run in one lane of a capillary gel, and read with a laser detector. This advance allows for more accurate sequence reading while using less time and reagents (**Fig. 7**).

PYROSEQUENCING

Pyrosequencing is a method of DNA sequencing based on sequencing by the principle of synthesis. First, a sequencing primer is hybridized to a single-stranded DNA template in the presence of the enzymes, DNA polymerase, ATP sulfurylase, luciferase, and apyrase, and the substrates, adenosine 5′ phosphosulfate (APS) and luciferin.[13–15]

The first of 4 dNTPs are then added to the reaction and DNA polymerase incorporates it only if it is complementary to the base in the template strand. Each incorporation event is accompanied by the release of pyrophosphate (PPi) in a quantity equimolar to the amount of incorporated nucleotide (**Fig. 8**, step 2).

ATP sulfurylase quantitatively converts PPi to ATP in the presence of APS. This ATP drives the luciferase-mediated conversion of luciferin to oxyluciferin, which generates visible light in amounts proportional to the ATP generated. The light produced in the luciferase-catalyzed reaction is detected by a charge-coupled device camera and seen as a peak in a Pyrogram. The height of each peak is proportional to the number of a specific nucleotide incorporated (**Fig. 8**, step 3).

Apyrase, a nucleotide degrading enzyme, continuously degrades ATP and unincorporated dNTPs. Apyrase switches off the light-promoting reaction and regenerates the reaction solution. The next dNTP is then added (**Fig. 8**, step 4).

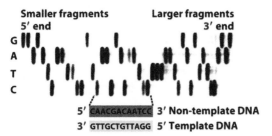

Fig. 6. Classic Sanger sequence film with representative sample sequence. (*Adapted from* Freeman S. Biological science. 2nd edition. Upper Saddle River, NJ: Pearson Education, Inc.; 2005. p. 410; with permission.)

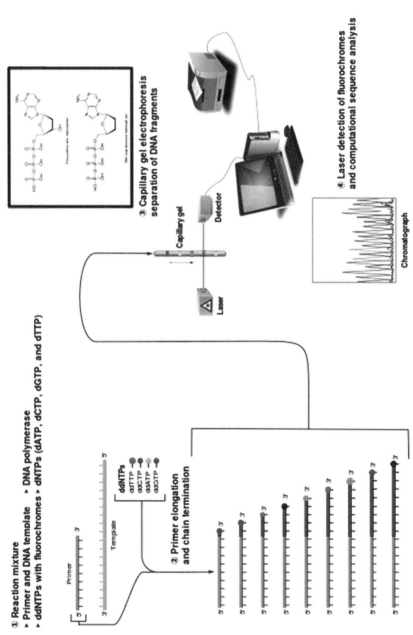

Fig. 7. Next Gen Sanger sequencing using only one tube and fluorescent-labeled ddNTPs.

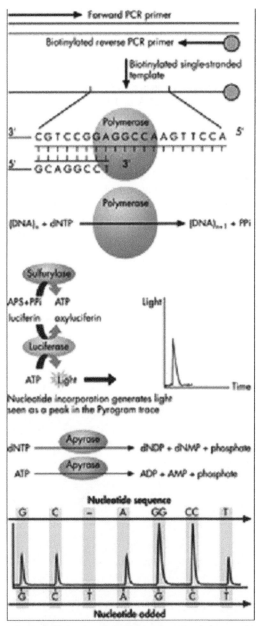

Fig. 8. Stepwise illustration of the pyrosequencing method. (Image kindly provided by © QIAGEN all rights reserved.)

The addition of dNTPs is performed one at a time (G then C then T then A then G then C then T, etc). As the process continues, the cDNA strand is built up and the nucleotide sequence is determined from the signal peaks in the Pyrogram (**Fig. 8**, Step 5).

Deoxyadenosine alpha-thiotriphosphate is used as a substitute for dATP because it is used efficiently by DNA polymerase, but is not recognized by luciferase (all figures from describing pyrosequencing adapted from http://www.adelaide.edu.au/saef/new/whatis/).

DENATURING GRADIENT GEL ELECTROPHORESIS

Denaturing gradient gel electrophoresis is a widespread technique that can be used to separate similar sized fragments of DNA or RNA based on the composition of the double-stranded fragments. The melting temperature (ie, the temperature at which base pairs in a dsDNA fragment lose their bond) depends on the base-pair composition of a fragment. Even in the case of a one base-pair substitution, the fragment will melt at a different temperature.[16]

By adding a GC-rich tail (called a GC clamp) to one of the primers for the amplification, a fragment is produced that will only partially melt when it is run into a denaturing gradient gel. The GC clamp will remain double stranded, which causes the fragment to stop migrating when it reaches a certain point in the gel. This process will occur at a different position in the gel when one or more base pairs are substituted, deleted, or inserted. Therefore, allelic variation or mutation can be detected (**Fig. 9**) using this method.[17] Clinically, Denaturing Gradient Gel Electrophoresis (DGGE) could be used to confirm the presence of and distinguish between which types of mycobacteria are present in a sample.[18] It can also be used to determine what mutations exist in BRCA1 and BRCA2 genes of an individual.[19]

In this method, the gradient is typically a urea and formamide (UF) gradient. The use of the UF gradient results in the ability to run the gel at a much lower temperature than

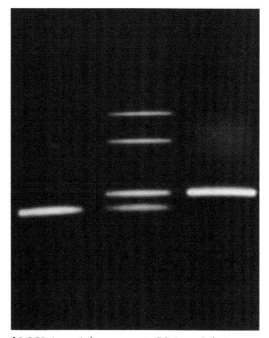

Fig. 9. Illustration of DGGE. Lane 1: homozygous GC. Lane 2: heterozygous sample. Lane 3: homozygous AT. (*Courtesy of* Dr R.W.M. Hofstra, Department of Medical Genetics, University of Groningen, The Netherlands.)

without, using the gradient. A 10% increase in UF concentration has the same effect as a 3.2°C increase in temperature.

HIGH-RESOLUTION MELTING ANALYSIS

High-resolution melting analysis (HRM) is a technique for fast, high-throughput post-PCR analysis of genetic mutations or variance in nucleic acid sequences. It enables researchers to detect and categorize genetic mutations rapidly (eg, SNPs), identify new genetic variants without sequencing (gene scanning), or determine the genetic variation in a population (eg, viral diversity) before sequencing.

The first step of the HRM protocol is the amplification of the region of interest, using standard PCR techniques, in the presence of a specialized dsDNA binding dye (such as SYBR Green). This specialized dye is highly fluorescent when bound to dsDNA and poorly fluorescent in the unbound state. This change allows the user to monitor the DNA amplification during PCR (as in real-time or quantitative PCR).

After completion of the PCR step, a high-resolution melt curve is produced by increasing the temperature of the PCR product, typically in increments of 0.008 to 0.2°C, thereby gradually denaturing an amplified DNA target. Because SYBR Green is only fluorescent when bound to dsDNA, fluorescence decreases as duplex DNA is denatured, which produces a characteristic melting profile; this is termed melting analysis. The melting profile depends on the length, GC content, sequence, and heterozygosity of the amplified target. When set up correctly, HRM is sensitive enough to allow the detection of a single base change between otherwise identical nucleotide sequences.[20,21]

SOUTHERN AND NORTHERN HYBRIDIZATIONS

Both Southern and Northern hybridizations combine electrophoretic separation of test nucleic acid with transfer to a solid support and subsequent hybridization. These assays, therefore, not only give information about the presence of hybridization but also permit determination of the molecular weight of the hybridizing species.

The original procedure was termed Southern blot hybridization or Southern blotting, after its inventor, E. M. Southern. In this assay, the sample is DNA. Northern blotting was named by analogy for the technique using RNA samples. (Extending the analogy even further, the Western blot is a similar procedure in which proteins are subjected to electrophoresis and transfer; a Southwestern blot has been described for a technique separating and blotting DNA followed by incubation with protein solutions to permit evaluation of specific DNA-binding proteins.)

Sample preparation is time-consuming and labor intensive for both of these techniques. Degradation of sample nucleic acids is not tolerated by the assays, and a relatively large amount of starting material is required. For Southern hybridizations, the DNA must be purified with minimal shearing because sizing of the DNA fragments is achieved through digestion with one or more restriction enzymes. Shearing and degradation introduce random breaks in the sample, reducing the quantity available to be cut specifically at appropriate recognition sequences. Impurities in the sample may interfere with the activity and sequence specificity of the restriction enzyme. Partially or improperly digested samples can produce spurious band sizes or result in such a reduced concentration of the specific band that it is no longer detected during hybridization. For Northern hybridizations, the starting material is RNA, and extreme care must be taken to avoid degradation during sample collection and preparation because of the ubiquitous nature of RNases. RNA is composed of fragment sizes determined by transcription and processing of message and ribosomal RNA. It is not digested before electrophoresis, but is separated under denaturing conditions to remove secondary structure.

The size-separated fragments in the agarose gel are then transferred to a nylon or nitrocellulose membrane. As originally designed, the transfer occurred passively through capillary action. Most current applications use vacuum or pressure to speed the transfer. After transfer, baking or ultraviolet cross-linking immobilizes the nucleic acids and the entire membrane is then hybridized with labeled probe under stringent conditions.

Hybridization is followed by autoradiographic, colorimetric, or chemiluminescent detection of bands that are bound to the probe. Interpretation involves both detection of a hybridizing species and determination of the molecular weight of the molecule. These technically demanding assays require several days to perform but may be required in clinical applications in which the information cannot be obtained in any other format. The presence of bands at molecular weights different from normal or germline (developmentally unaltered) samples can indicate a change in the genetic material.[22–25]

RESTRICTION FRAGMENT LENGTH POLYMORPHISM ANALYSIS

Restriction fragment length polymorphism (RFLP) analysis is a method that uses restriction endonuclease digestion of DNA and gel electrophoretics separation of the resulting fragments (**Fig. 10**). This technique allows the study of small variances called polymorphisms that occur in the DNA sequences between individuals of the same species. These variances occur in the form of differing numbers of small sequence repeats of DNA—called tandem repeats, minisatellites, and microsatellites—that are normally found in the noncoding regions of DNA. Polymorphisms can occur as a result of mutations—deletions, inversions, additions, substitutions, and translocations—to the DNA sequence.

Briefly, DNA is carefully isolated (so as to cause as little degradation and mechanical fragmentation as possible) and then digested with a particular endonuclease. The digested DNA is electrophoretically separated in an agarose gel. At this point the separated DNA samples can be viewed using DNA binding dyes, such as ethidium bromide, to compare the banding patterns. Alternatively, the DNA fragments can be Southern blotted (see above), hybridized with labeled probes, and then analyzed.

Therefore, if one were to digest DNA from 2 individuals (excluding identical twins and clones) and separate the resulting fragments by gel electrophoresis, some differences may be found in the 2 resulting banding patterns because of the differing number of tandem repeats between restriction sites from one individual to another. Analysis of the banding of an individual yields what is commonly known as a "genetic fingerprint."

Using RFLP analysis, one may also observe a difference in the RFLP patterns between normal and diseased tissue (ie, tumor) from the same individual. If a tumor results from a genetic alteration (mutation), that alteration may result in a change in the size of one or more bands as a result of additions or deletions of DNA. In addition, single-nucleotide alterations may be observable via RFLP analysis if the alteration occurs within the sequence of just one of the endonuclease restriction sites, rendering that particular site unrecognizable to and uncut by the enzyme, which ultimately changes the banding pattern.[26]

REVERSE LINE-BLOT HYBRIDIZATION

Reverse line-blot hybridization, also called "spacer oligonucleotide typing" (spoligo-typing),[27] is a method that can detect and identify pathogens based on the presence

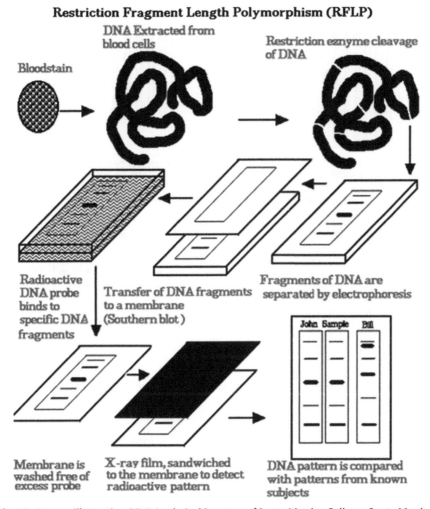

Restriction Fragment Length Polymorphism (RFLP)

DNA Extracted from blood cells

Restriction eznyme cleavage of DNA

Bloodstain

Radioactive DNA probe binds to specific DNA fragments

Transfer of DNA fragments to a membrane (Southern blot)

Fragments of DNA are separated by electrophoresis

John Sample Bill

Membrane is washed free of excess probe

X-ray film, sandwiched to the membrane to detect radioactive pattern

DNA pattern is compared with patterns from known subjects

Fig. 10. Process illustrating RFLP Analysis. (*Courtesy of* Santa Monica College, Santa Monica, CA; with permission.)

and comparison of pathogen-specific genes and is useful for confirming the presence of specific pathogens and a proper course of treatment based on possible multidrug resistance. For example, wild-type *M tuberculosis* is a slow-growing bacterium, requiring 2 to 6 weeks to culture, and is sensitive to treatment with rifampicin (RIF). Mutations in the *rpoB* gene can render it resistant to RIF. Using this information, the mutation hot-spot region of the *rpoB* gene is first amplified by mpPCR using as many as 20 different biotinylated primers, which yield labeled amplified products.[28] The PCR products are hybridized to a set of wild-type and mutant oligonucleotide probes, which are covalently bound to a membrane, by reverse line blotting (**Fig. 11**). It is called "reverse" because, in contrast to Southern or Northern blotting where the sample is transferred onto a membrane and then probed, the probe is first systematically bound to the membrane and the sample is then hybridized to it.

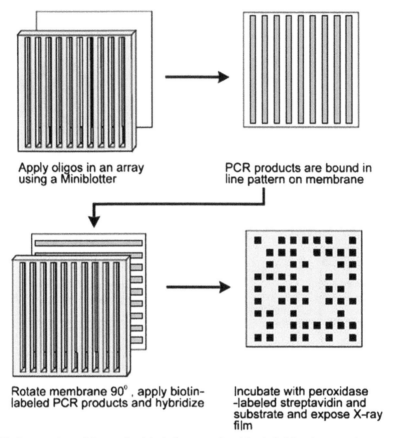

Apply oligos in an array
using a Miniblotter

PCR products are bound in
line pattern on membrane

Rotate membrane 90°, apply biotin-
labeled PCR products and hybridize

Incubate with peroxidase
-labeled streptavidin and
substrate and expose X-ray
film

Fig. 11. Preparation of the probe-labeled reverse line-blot hybridization membrane.

Positive hybridization is detected on film after streptavidin-peroxidase incubation and enhanced chemiluminescence. RIF-sensitive strains only hybridize with the wild-type probes, whereas resistant strains will fail to hybridize with one or more wild-type probes and show additional hybridization signals for the mutant probes (**Fig. 12**). The resultant hybridization pattern elucidates the genotype of the M tuberculosis and thus a proper treatment protocol.

HYBRID CAPTURE

Hybrid capture is a nucleic acid hybridization technology that can precede signal amplification and often uses fluorophore or chemiluminescent detection. To date, human papillomavirus (HPV) cannot be cultured in vitro, and immunologic tests are inadequate to determine the presence of HPV cervical infection. Indirect evidence of anogenital HPV infection can be obtained through physical examination and by the presence of characteristic cellular changes associated with viral replication in Papanicolaou smear or biopsy specimens. Alternately, biopsies can be analyzed by nucleic acid hybridization to detect the presence of HPV DNA directly. In the case of modern molecular-based HPV tests, specimens containing the target DNA hybridize with a specific HPV RNA probe cocktail. The resultant RNA:DNA

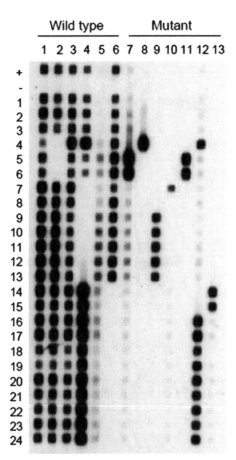

Fig. 12. Results of a reverse line-blot hybridization assay.

hybrids are captured onto the surface of a solid media (ie, a microplate well coated with antibodies specific for RNA:DNA hybrids or covalently linked to beads). Immobilized hybrids are then reacted with alkaline phosphatase–conjugated antibodies specific for the RNA:DNA hybrids and detected with a chemiluminescent substrate.

Several alkaline phosphatase molecules are conjugated to each antibody. Multiple conjugated antibodies bind to each captured hybrid, resulting in substantial signal amplification. As the substrate is cleaved by the bound alkaline phosphatase, light is emitted that is measured as relative light units on a luminometer (**Fig. 13**). The intensity of the light emitted denotes the presence or absence of target DNA in the specimen.[29] In the case of HPV, although this technique can elucidate the presence and load of the virus, it cannot determine which specific types of HPV are present. For the identification of the HPV strains present in the sample, PCR with HPV strain–specific primers would be required.[30]

BRANCHED DNA ASSAYS

In contrast with techniques that rely on PCR, the sensitivity of branched DNA (bDNA) methods is achieved by signal amplification on the bDNA probe after direct binding of

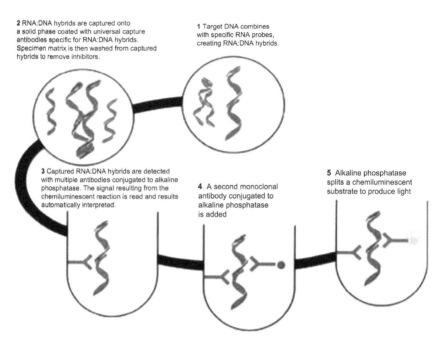

2 RNA:DNA hybrids are captured onto a solid phase coated with universal capture antibodies specific for RNA:DNA hybrids. Specimen matrix is then washed from captured hybrids to remove inhibitors.

1 Target DNA combines with specific RNA probes, creating RNA:DNA hybrids.

3 Captured RNA:DNA hybrids are detected with multiple antibodies conjugated to alkaline phosphatase. The signal resulting from the chemiluminescent reaction is read and results automatically interpreted.

4 A second monoclonal antibody conjugated to alkaline phosphatase is added

5 Alkaline phosphatase splits a chemiluminescent substrate to produce light

Fig. 13. Hybrid capture test principle. (Image kindly provided by © QIAGEN all rights reserved.)

a large hybridization complex to the RNA target sequence. This series of hybridization steps results in a "sandwich" complex of probes and target sequence. These unusual synthetic oligonucleotides are composed of a primary sequence and secondary sequences that result in a branched structure extending from the primary sequence.

There is no synthesis reaction taking place. However, there are 2 steps to this assay: the capturing step and the signal amplification step. In the capturing step there are 2 capturing oligonucleotide probes: the capture probe and the capture extender probe. The capture probe is linked to the bottom of a microwell plate much like the one used in hybrid capture. The capture extender probe will hybridize to both the capture probe and a specific sequence on the target RNA, effectively anchoring it to the solid medium (bottom of the microwell plate). The assay then continues to the signal amplification step whereby label extender probes are hybridized to specific sequences at precise distances from each other on the target RNA. The label extender probes are designed to serve as platforms for hybridization to preamplifier probes, which only remain attached if hybridized to 2 adjacent label extender probes. Next, amplifier probes, oligonucleotides labeled with alkaline phosphatase, are hybridized to the preamplifier probes. Finally, the assay is treated with a chemoreactive substrate that facilitates the chemiluminescent reaction and is read by a luminometer. This assay can be multiplexed by linking the capture probe to beads instead of the surface of a microwell (**Fig. 14**).

The signal in the bDNA assay is proportional to the number of alkaline phosphatase–labeled probes that hybridize to bDNA secondary sequences. As such, the target RNA can be blocked with blocking probes to increase the stringency of the primary probes bound to it. As with all chemiluminescent-based assays of this type, quantification is achieved by establishing a standard curve as well as negative and positive controls for each run.[31]

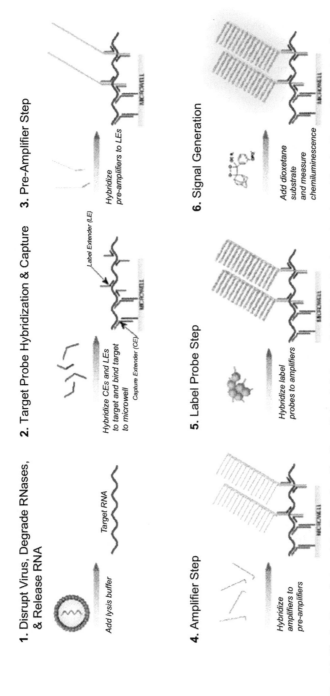

Fig. 14. Illustration of virus detection using the Qauntiplex 3.0 Assay via bDNA technology developed by the Bayer Corporation. (*From* Campas M, Katakis I. DNA biochip arraying, detection and amplification strategies. Trends Analyt Chem 2004;23(1):49–62; with permission.)

IN SITU HYBRIDIZATION

In situ hybridization is simply the detection of specific genetic information within a morphologic context.[32] In situ hybridization facilitates simultaneous detection, localization, and quantification of individual DNA or RNA molecules at the cellular level in a fixed sample using labeled oligonucleotides or peptides as probes. This specialized type of solid-support assay involves taking morphologically intact tissue, cells, or chromosomes affixed to a glass microscope slide through the hybridization process. Briefly, after a tissue sample is fixed, it is permeabilized and labeled probes are added and allowed to hybridize to target molecules. The samples are then washed and viewed using bright-field or fluorescent microscopy.

Autoradiographic, chromogenic[33] (CISH), and fluorescent (FISH) methods of detection have been applied. Evaluation of the final product is analogous to evaluation of immunohistochemistry and requires experience in histopathology. The strength of the method lies in linking microscopic morphologic evaluation with detection via hybridization.

The method also has applications in cytogenetic analysis of metaphase chromosome spreads or of interphase nuclei. In this context, the detection is usually accomplished via FISH. Detecting numerical aberrations or translocations of chromosomes can be achieved rapidly using probes for specific targets. FISH avoids some of the difficulties of conventional cytogenetics and may have greater sensitivity for some targets. Although FISH cannot completely replace karyotyping, it can complement and reduce the need for the frequency of cytogenetic analysis.[34]

Newer variations of FISH and CISH are exploiting the possibilities of automation (fast-FISH) and expanding the information that can be obtained in a single assay. FICTION (Fluorescence Immunophenotyping and Interphase Cytogenetics as a Tool for Investigation Of Neoplasms) combines immunophenotyping with FISH; GOLDFISH (Gold-Facilitated In Situ Hybridization) is a gold-enhanced bright field chromogenic in situ gene amplification assay,[35] and fiber FISH makes it possible to detect and map chromosomal break points simultaneously. In situ hybridization can be very labor intensive and tedious and, because of the extremely labile nature of mRNA, gives inconsistent results for molecular diagnostic purposes. However, recent improvements resulting in automated processing of slides through the assay hold much promise for more widespread adoption of this technique.

Other Technologies

Microarray-based technologies have the capacity to interrogate tens of thousands of genes at one time. As such, although array-based algorithms have been FDA approved in selective cases (p450 cytochrome oxidase), the application of the clinical marketplace is not well defined. Array-based methods can be found elsewhere[36]; however, time will determine how such methods are to be interpreted, reported to the physician, and ultimately, used for effective patient management.

REFERENCES

1. Saiki RK, Gelfand DH, Stoffel S, et al. Primer-directed enzymatic amplification of DNA with a thermostable DNA polymerase. Science 1988;239:487–91.
2. Myers TW, Gelfand DH. Reverse transcription and DNA amplification by a Thermus thermophilus DNA polymerase. Biochemistry 1991;30:7661–6.
3. Heid CA, Stevens J, Livak KJ, et al. Real time quantitativePCR. Genome Res 1996;6:986–94.

4. VanGuilder HD, Vrana KE, Freeman WM. Twenty-five years of quantitative PCR for gene expression analysis. Biotechniques 2008;44(5):619–26.
5. Spackman E, Suarez DL. Type A influenza virus detection and quantitation by real-time RT-PCR. Methods Mol Biol 2008;436:19–26.
6. Chamberlain JS, Gibbs RA, Ranier JE, et al. Deletion screening of the Duchenne muscular dystrophy locus via multiplex DNA amplification. Nucleic Acids Res 1988;16(23):11141–56.
7. Merante F, Yaghoubian S, Janeczko R. Principles of the xTAG respiratory viral panel assay. J Clin Virol 2007;40:S31–5.
8. Walker GT, Little M, Nadeau J, et al. Strand displacement amplification—an isothermal, in vitro DNA amplification technique. Nucleic Acids Res 1992;20: 1691–6.
9. Walker GT, Little MC, Nadeau JG, et al. Isothermal in vitro amplification of DNA by a restriction enzyme/DNA polymerase system. Proc Natl Acad Sci U S A 1992;89: 392–6.
10. Walker GT. Empirical aspects of strand displacement amplification [review]. PCR Methods Appl 1993;3(1):1–6.
11. Down JA, O'Connell MA, Dey MS, et al. Detection of Mycobacterium tuberculosis in respiratory specimens by strand displacement amplification of DNA. J Clin Microbiol 1996;34(4):860–5.
12. Available at: http://www.gen-probe.com/science/#technologies-0.
13. Ronaghi M, Uhlén M, Nyrén P. A sequencing method based on real-time pyrophosphate. Science 1998;281(5375):363.
14. Nyrén P. The history of pyrosequencing. Methods Mol Biol 2007;373:1–14.
15. Nordstrom T, Ronaghi M, Forsberg L, et al. Direct analysis of single-nucleotide polymorphism on double-stranded DNA by pyrosequencing. Biotechnol Appl Biochem 2000;31:107–12.
16. Fischer SG, Lerman LS. DNA fragments differing by single base-pair substitutions are separated in denaturing gradient gels: correspondence with melting theory. Proc Natl Acad Sci U S A 1983;80(6):1579–83.
17. Available at: http://www.ingeny.com/htdocs/DGGE.html.
18. McAuliffe L, Ellis Richard J, Lawes Jo R, et al. 16S rDNA PCR and denaturing gradient gel electrophoresis; a single generic test for detecting and differentiating Mycoplasma species. J Med Microbiol 2005;54:731–9.
19. van der Hout Annemarie H, van den Ouweland Ans MW, van der Luijt Rob B, et al. A DGGE system for comprehensive mutation screening of BRCA1 and BRCA2: application in a Dutch cancer clinic setting. Hum Mutat 2006;27(7):654–66.
20. Ririe K, Rasmussen RP, Wittwer CT. Product differentiation by analysis of DNA melting curves during the polymerase chain reaction. Anal Biochem 1997;245: 154–60.
21. Available at: http://www.kapabiosystems.com/public/pdfs/kapa-hrm-fast-pcrkits/Introduction_to_High_Resolution_Melt _Analysis_Guide.pdf.
22. Alberts B, Johnson A, Lewis J, et al. Molecular biology of the cell. 5th edition. New York: Garland Science, Taylor & Francis Group; 2008. p. 538–9.
23. Southern EM. Detection of specific sequences among DNA fragments separated by gel electrophoresis. J Mol Biol 1975;98(3):503–17.
24. Alwine JC, Kemp DJ, Stark GR. Method for detection of specific RNAs in agarose gels by transfer to diazobenzyloxymethyl-paper and hybridization with DNA probes. Proc Natl Acad Sci U S A 1977;74(12):5350–4.
25. Kevil CG, Walsh L, Laroux FS, et al. An improved, rapid northern protocol. Biochem Biophys Res Commun 1997;238:277–9.

26. Rosetti S, Englisch S, Bresin E, et al. Detection of mutations in human genes by a new rapid method: cleavage fragment length polymorphism analysis (CFLPA). Mol Cell Probes 1997;11:155–60.

27. Molhuizen HO, Bunschoten AE, Schouls LM, et al. Rapid detection and simultaneous strain differentiation of Mycobacterium tuberculosis complex bacteria by spoligotyping. Methods Mol Biol 1998;101:381–94.

28. Cowan LS, Diem L, Brake MC, et al. Transfer of a Mycobacterium tuberculosis genotyping method, spoligotyping, from a reverse line-blot hybridization, membrane-based assay to the luminex multianalyte profiling system. J Clin Microbiol 2004;42(1):474–7.

29. Poljak M, Brenčič A, Seme K, et al. Comparative evaluation of first- and second-generation digene hybrid capture assays for detection of human papillomaviruses associated with high or intermediate risk for cervical cancer. J Clin Microbiol 1999;37(3):796–7.

30. Available at: http://www.thehpvtest.com/~/media/5C4BD0982BED4E3788F65B36AF829AAD.ashx.

31. Collins ML, Zayati C, Detmer JJ, et al. Preparation and characterization of RNA standards for use in quantitative branched-DNA hybridization assays. Anal Biochem 1995;226:120–9.

32. Gall JG, Pardue ML. Formation and detection of RNA-DNA hybrid molecules in cytological preparations. Proc Natl Acad Sci U S A 1969;63(2):378–83.

33. Tautz D, Pfeifle C. A non-radioactive in situ hybridization method for the localization of specific RNAs in Drosophila embryos reveals translational control of the segmentation gene hunchback. Chromosoma 1989;98(2):81–5.

34. Jin L, Lloyd RV. In situ hybridization: methods and applications. J Clin Lab Anal 1997;11(1):2–9.

35. Tubbs R, Pettay J, Skacel M, et al. Gold-facilitated in situ hybridization: a brightfield autometallographic alternative to fluorescence in situ hybridization for detection of HER-2/neu gene amplification. Am J Pathol 2002;160:1589–95.

36. Bluth MH. Hybridization array technologies in McPherson and Pincus: Henry's clinical diagnosis and management by laboratory methods. 22nd edition. New York: Saunders Publishing; 2011. p. 1282–9.

Clinical Implication of MicroRNAs in Molecular Pathology

Seema Sethi, MD[a], Shadan Ali, MS[b], Dejuan Kong, PhD[c],
Philip A. Philip, MD, PhD[d], Fazlul H. Sarkar, PhD[e,f],*

KEYWORDS

- miRNAs • Fine-needle aspirates • Serum • Pancreatic cancer • Prostate cancer

KEY POINTS

- The miRNAs have immense potential in the clinical arena because they can be detected in the blood; serum; tissues (fresh and formalin fixed paraffin embedded); and also fine-needle aspirate specimens.
- Identification of novel molecular miRNAs and their target oncogenomic signatures have the potential to significantly impact clinical management.
- Incorporating miRNA expression profiling on tissue samples in the future may not only confirm diagnosis categorizing diseases and their subtypes but also may predict drug response in helping clinicians define the precise therapy to each individual.
- Increasing the knowledge of disease progression and tumor recurrence might also improve the development of personalized therapies.
- The most attractive feature of miRNA-based therapy is that a single miRNA could be useful for targeting multiple genes that are deregulated in cancers, which can be further investigated through systems biology and network analysis that will allow designing cancer-specific personalized therapy.

The authors have nothing to disclose.
[a] Department of Pathology, Karmanos Cancer Institute, Wayne State University School of Medicine, 4100 John R Street, Detroit, MI 48201, USA; [b] Department of Oncology, Karmanos Cancer Institute, Wayne State University School of Medicine, 703 Hudson Webber Cancer Research Center, 4100 John R Street, Detroit, MI 48201, USA; [c] Department of Pathology, Karmanos Cancer Institute, Wayne State University School of Medicine, 715 Hudson Webber Cancer Research Center, 4100 John R Street, Detroit, MI 48201, USA; [d] Department of Oncology, Karmanos Cancer Institute, Wayne State University School of Medicine, 4 Hudson Webber Cancer Research Center, 4100 John R Street, Detroit, MI 48201, USA; [e] Department of Pathology, Karmanos Cancer Institute, Wayne State University School of Medicine, 740 Hudson Webber Cancer Research Center, 4100 John R Street, Detroit, MI 48201, USA; [f] Department of Oncology, Karmanos Cancer Institute, Wayne State University School of Medicine, 4100 John R Street, Detroit, MI 48201, USA
* Corresponding author. Department of Pathology, Karmanos Cancer Institute, Wayne State University School of Medicine, 740 Hudson Webber Cancer Research Center, 4100 John R Street, Detroit, MI 48201.
E-mail address: fsarkar@med.wayne.edu

Clin Lab Med 33 (2013) 773–786
http://dx.doi.org/10.1016/j.cll.2013.08.001
0272-2712/13/$ – see front matter © 2013 Elsevier Inc. All rights reserved.

INTRODUCTION

In this era of personalized medicine, a plethora of molecular markers are emerging to be used as novel tools in molecular pathology. The role of the pathologist is no longer confined to being behind the glass slide. Rapid advances in the fields of molecular biology and medicine have led to the development of the newly maturing field of molecular pathology, which has ramifications for the therapeutic management of patients. This field incorporates the use of cellular molecules in the clinical arena for early and accurate diagnosis, determining prognosis and risk stratification of disease, as therapeutic targets for designing molecular therapies, disease surveillance, and more recently prevention of disease progression and metastasis.

The field of molecular pathology has revolutionized clinical medicine. It further directs to the development of a novel branch of molecular pharmacotherapeutics. This is a newly developed branch of pharmacology that evaluates the impact of human genetic variations, which affect individual drug responses and further analyzes mechanisms to overcome drug resistance and tailor pharmacologic drug response based on molecular alterations within cells. It includes the potential and challenges of drug optimization, the implications for drug development and regulation, ethical and social aspects of pharmacogenomics, signal transduction, the use of knockout mice, and informed consent process in pharmacogenetic research. Based on gene expression patterns seen in different tumors in individualized patients the tumor is classified into different genotypes and treated based on an independent set of molecular and genetic characteristics.[1] This molecular tumor profile is then used to select specific targeted treatment approaches for patients with specific types of cancer.[2] Furthermore, the response to molecular-based therapy is then evaluated taking into consideration the patients' individual drug response and drug resistance of the tumor cells if any, and methods to overcome the same are explored.[3]

Recent literature reveals a deluge of several small molecule inhibitors with possible clinical use in future clinical trials.[4,5] However, before they can be brought into the clinical arena there is an ongoing process of drug evaluation in vitro and in animal models. This has resulted in significant expansion of the responsibilities of the pathologist in identifying druggable targets, prognostic biomarkers, histopathologic risk predictors, and further assisting in developing molecular targeted therapies. It is in the realm of the pathologist to identify these small molecules, which can be targeted through these small molecule inhibitors. After the small molecular alterations are identified in a subset of tumor types, these are stratified by the pathologist into those that develop early in the course of carcinogenesis making them relevant biomarkers of disease identification for early and accurate diagnosis. Additionally, the pathologist evaluates whether these small molecules can be used in risk stratification and to determine prognosis in specific tumors. Furthermore, the pathologist can assist in the drug trials in determining the efficacy of small molecule inhibitors in reducing the size of the tumor, reducing the number of tumor cells, and the overall tumor burden leading to pathologic and microscopic identification of druggable target molecules.

One recently described class of molecule that is showing far-reaching clinical effects in molecular pathology is that encompassing microRNA (miRNA) biology and technology.[6,7] These are small, noncoding endogenous single-stranded RNAs comprising only 19 to 25 nucleotides in length but on average of about 22 nucleotides in length.[6,7] First described in 1993, these molecules are actively comprised in the regulation of multiple physiologic and pathologic procedures in humans, animals, and plants. They regulate the physiologic embryonic stem cell differentiation[7,8] and recent studies have also demonstrated their key roles in the pathogenetic evolution, progression, and metastasis of carcinomas.[9–11]

The proposed mechanism of action of miRNAs is through the posttranscriptional gene expression regulation through the 3'-untranslated region binding of target mRNAs.[7,8] This causes mRNA degradation or suppression of their translation to functional proteins.[4] Transcripts complementary to the 3'-untranslated region govern the translation by the RNA-RNA interaction. This results in the translational suppression or cleavage of the targeted mRNA because of the damaged complementarity between micro and messenger RNA. The miRNA genes transcript occurs by RNA polymerase II or III, which then yield primary miRNA. The location of maximum miRNA genes is in intergenic regions about 1 kilobase away from annotated genes.[7,8]

In addition to general transcriptional regulation of mRNA expression and translation, miRNAs also influence the development, progression, and metastasis of cancers.[6–8,12–14] Their functional effect may differ depending on their expression levels. They have either an oncogenic potential or tumor suppressor effect depending on their downstream impact on target genes and thereby controlling the biologic manifestations of cancers.

Emerging evidence suggests that cancer stem cells (CSCs) and epithelial-to-mesenchymal transition phenotypic cells are regulated by the expression of miRNAs, implicating their role in chemoresistance and cancer metastasis.[15–17] There is evidence that these molecules are critical in the formation of CSCs making them potential targets for overcoming drug resistance. Additionally, they have been proposed to have a part in the epithelial-to-mesenchymal transition phenomenon with implications in cancer drug resistance and metastasis.[17]

CLINICAL PERSPECTIVE

Cancers are a common clinical problem worldwide leading to immense mortality, morbidity, and escalating health care costs. Despite rapid technologic and clinical advances, the cancer-related mortality and morbidity remain high, which also impacts patients' quality of life. Recent advances in the imaging and diagnostic modalities have resulted in early diagnosis of many cancers wherein select treatments have led to miraculous results with significant reduction in patient anguish. However, many malignancies still remain occult until they have reached the late stages of the disease or have metastasized. The best of treatment options including multimodal therapeutic approaches have yielded minimal success in such instances. This underlines the need to use novel technologic advances in molecular biology from bench to patient bedside for clinical patient management. Moreover, the molecular mechanism of carcinogenesis, progression, and metastasis in some cancers is still largely unknown despite the "omic" revolution, which clearly suggests that further development in the areas of molecular signatures of disease aggressiveness is urgently needed.

Rapid progress occurring in technology and knowledge of molecular pathology has prompted a paradigm shift in the therapeutic patient management in the clinical arena. There is evidence of increasing integration of molecular markers with clinical and morphologic disease criteria to yield clinically relevant diagnostic, prognostic, and therapeutic algorithms for patient management. Moreover, selection of molecular targeted therapies and determination of prognosis and risk stratification of patients are being based on genomic and proteomic molecular diagnostic and prognostic signatures for patient care.

There is a unique opportunity to think outside the box and look at clinical problems in an analytical manner to solve cancer research dilemmas for the ultimate benefit of patients. Newly developed high throughput, quantitative image-based methodologies for analysis and subcellular identification of alteration in cancers hold extreme promise in this regard. However, before these can be clinically applicable, they need to be correlated with the morphologic and clinical findings.

Cellular molecules, such as miRNAs, have an immense potential in the clinical realm of molecular pathology. Furthermore, one particular miRNA may target multiple genes in a context-dependent manner, suggesting that targeted deregulation of one miRNA will have effects on multiple targets, which seems to be an attractive attributes for cancer therapy. Therefore, modulating miRNAs activity may provide openings for novel cancer interventions. They have widespread clinical application in different aspects of patient care because their expression levels vary in different tumors and also alter with the disease progression.

Several miRNAs with oncogenic potential have been demonstrated to be upregulated in cancers and miRNAs with tumor-suppressive effect are downregulated in malignancies. Translating the application of miRNAs in clinical context has been enhanced by the applicability of several novel high throughput multiplex technologies on a wide variety of patient samples including blood; serum; tissues (fresh and formalin-fixed paraffin embedded); and cerebrospinal fluid.[12,13,18–20] Apart from being able to decipher small molecules, these technologies lower laboratory costs, increase operational productivity, and enhance yield.[21–24] These are an integral part of the clinical armamentarium of the new age pathologist, which has strengthened diagnostic capabilities in the move forward into the era of precision medicine.

Therapeutic decision-making and patient clinical management in the current clinical practice is being dictated more by alterations occurring in the tumor microenvironment at the molecular level namely genetic, epigenetic, miRNA, and multispectral protein levels than by the histomorphologic spectrum alone. This has led to a multisystem approach to a patient that includes a team composed of several clinicians with expertise in medical, surgical, pathology, molecular biology, and pharmacotherapeutics working together in synergy for the maximum benefit of the patient minimizing the side effects and using drugs with targeted approach to achieve the goal of personalized medicine.

USE OF MOLECULAR PATHOLOGY PRACTICE

Molecular diagnostic applications are now an integral part of the management algorithms of several solid tumors. With the use of molecular diagnostics in oncology, pathologists hope to assist early and accurate diagnosis of malignant disease processes during initial work-up. Molecular diagnostics can also help in risk stratification based on molecular parameters. Additionally, one can use the molecular biomarkers for disease surveillance during treatment and follow-up. Emerging evidence directed to the complex molecular changes involved in the development and progression of different malignancies produced innovative diagnostic molecular tools leading to the introduction of targeted therapies. In lung cancer, miR-27a regulation of MET, EGFR, and Sprouty2 is being explored for targeted therapies.[25] The promising therapeutic targets for osteosarcoma patients include integrin, ezrin, statin, NOTCH/HES1, matrix metalloproteinases, and miR-215.[26] The miR-205BP/S3 is a possible promising therapeutic modality for melanoma.[27] The miR-34a may act as a tumor suppressor miRNA of hepatocellular carcinoma, and current efforts are under way to evaluate strategies to increase miR-34a level as a critical targeted therapy for hepatocellular carcinoma.[28]

Promising candidate biomarkers are being discovered that may soon switch to the realm of clinical management of malignancies. There is a need for new and improved molecular-based treatment options to improve on the modest outcome in patients with cancer. Prognostic molecular biomarkers require validation, which may be challenging at times, to help clinicians classify patients in need of early diagnosis. Recognizing predictive biomarkers that will stratify response to developing targeted therapeutics is additionally required arenas in cancer research and patient management. Furthermore, there is a need to identify clinically strong molecular tests to classify patients that are further responsive to certain drugs, in the early treatment design based on well-certified molecular prognosticators.

Scientific discoveries of molecular markers are often prematurely highlighted before the completion of clinical trials to establish appropriate application to disease. Before clinicians can use the molecular findings for clinical patient use there is a need for evidence-based guidelines established by knowledgeable clinicians to communicate emerging molecular clinical standards.

ROLE OF MIRNAS IN CLINICAL SPECIMENS

miRNA research has advanced within a decade from one publication to thousands of publications describing their role in gene regulation. miRNA expression profiling has been recently evaluated as a reliable diagnostic biomarker for differentiating between normal and tumor specimens.[6–8,12,29,30] It has shown to be deregulated in multiple cancers in human and mouse models, and has proved to play a critical role in the development and progression of the tumor.[6,7,12,29,30] Most of the miRNAs are differentially expressed, whereas some of them discriminate totally between normal and tumorigenic samples. The miRNA expression enhances (oncogenic miRNA) or reduces (tumor suppressor) as the tumor progresses and was found to be associated with drug resistance.[31]

This discovery of miRNA a decade ago, as a diagnostic and prognostic marker, has now led to miRNA-based targeted therapy in vitro, and may selectively predict better treatment outcome for patients with cancer. In addition, classification of an unknown tumor may be possible by the alteration of tumor-specific miRNA.[32] The nomenclature for assigning names to novel miRNAs for publication in peer-reviewed journals is done by miRBase, which is the central repository for miRNA sequence information.[33] It has an online database with all published miRNA sequences with links to the primary literature and to other secondary databases. Although some miRNAs are tumor specific,[32] miR-21 has proved to be the global oncogenic miRNA in many solid tumors.[34–39] The miRNAs with oncogenic potential include miR-155, miR-17-92, and miR-21[7] but it is not limited to these alone. The level of expression of miR-155 is upregulated in various carcinomas.[40–42] However, they are specifically significant in pancreatic cancers where they have prognostic relevance.[12,40,42,43]

Similarly, miRNA let-7 family and miR-200 family is frequently downregulated in many types of cancer, suggesting their role as a general tumor suppressor.[29,44–48] Low levels of let-7 miRNA[49] have been shown to have poorer prognosis with shorter postoperative survival in human lung cancer.[50] The tumor suppressor miR-34 is directly transactivated and induced by p53 signaling in the inhibition of human pancreatic cancer tumor-initiating cells.[51] Based on a recent literature review, it has been suggested that modulation of miRNAs is a novel molecular targeted therapeutic approach for cancer in vivo.[52] This has led to the development of an emerging field of miRNA pharmacotherapeutics, which involves altering the expression of miRNAs, which can inhibit cancer growth.[44] The therapeutic strategies suggested using miRNAs include the inhibition of upregulated miRNAs and re-expression of tumor suppressor miRNAs. They have also been shown to affect CSCs in overcoming drug resistance.[14] Regulation of miRNA levels in patients with ongoing cancer therapies would likely enhance the efficacy of their ongoing therapies.

Several synthetic small molecule inhibitors of miRNAs, such as chemically modified antisense oligonucleotides called "antagomiRs," are currently in use in vitro, targeting against specific oncogenic miRNAs. These antagomiRs silence the overexpressed oncogenic miRNAs in cancers by blocking their function.[7,30] In animal experiments, antagomiRs against miR-16, miR-122, miR-192, and miR-194 were found to be efficacious in reducing the levels of miRNA in the liver, lung, kidney, and ovaries.[52] Re-expression of tumor-suppressor miRNA, such as let-7, is another proposed miRNA therapeutic strategy to upregulate tumor-suppressor miRNA by exogenously transfecting with pre-let-7 that led to the inhibition of growth in vitro and in vivo.[15,44] These characteristics of miRNA suggest their potential role as novel biomarkers for diagnostic, prognostic, and therapeutic targets (**Fig. 1**).

METHODOLOGY AND CLINICAL IMPLICATIONS
Purification of miRNA from Human Plasma

The discovery of circulating miRNAs and their stability in plasma and serum is an interesting characteristic that could be used as noninvasive biomarkers for a variety of cancers, providing valuable tools to observe the changes during tumor progression.[29] Isolating miRNA of appropriate quality and quantity from blood is critical. Exosomal RNA seems to be the richest source of miRNA in the serum or plasma. We have successfully isolated RNA from plasma samples[29] and the detailed methodology is described next. Initially, the steps are carried out on ice, but later at room temperature. About 250 µL of plasma from each sample is centrifuged at 1000 × g for 5 minutes to

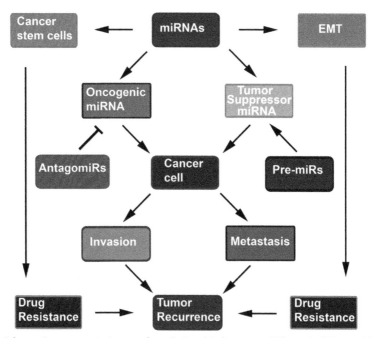

Fig. 1. Schematic representation on the relationship between CSCs and miRNAs with tumor aggressiveness, and the role of antagomiRs and pre-miRNAs on oncogenic and tumor suppressive miRNAs. EMT, epithelial-to-mesenchymal transition.

remove debris. The plasma is then transferred (200 μL) into a new tube along with 750 μL of QIAzol master mix containing 800 μL of QIAzol and 1 μg of MS2 RNA, and incubated for 5 minutes at room temperature. To this 200 μL of chloroform is added, mixed well, and incubated for 5 minutes at room temperature, followed by centrifugation at 12,000 × g for 15 minutes. All the subsequent steps are carried out at room temperature (20–25°C). The upper aqueous phase is moved into a new microtube containing 1.5 volume of ethanol. After mixing well, the solution is then transferred onto the RNeasy Mini Spin Column with about 750 μL each time, and centrifuged at 13,000 × g for 30 seconds. The flow-through is discarded, and the steps are repeated until the entire sample is used. The RNeasy Mini Column is then washed once with 700 μL of RWT, and three times with 500 μL RPE provided with the kit, and centrifuged for 13,000 × g for 1 minute. The flow-through is discarded each time. The RNA (containing miRNA) is eluted with about 25 μL of water in a new collection tube by centrifugation and stored at −80°C.

The amount of RNA obtained from blood is usually too low a yield compared with RNA obtained from tissue samples to be quantified using single-drop spectrophotometry technology (ie, Nanodrop). However, there are several miRNAs that are detectable in plasma or serum samples thus displaying the presence of miRNAs. One such miRNA is miR-21, which can be detected by conventional real-time reverse transcriptase polymerase chain reaction (RT-PCR) methodology, and is described next with significant modification using Exiqon-Universal cDNA synthesis kit (Exiqon, Woburn, MA).[12]

RT Reaction

The RT reaction is performed by using Exiqon-Universal cDNA synthesis kit. The cDNA for standard curve is synthesized by reverse transcription using the template mature miRNAs, which can be prepared by diluting it with water. The RT reaction is set up with 20 μL of sample containing 4 μL of 5× RT buffer, 2 μL of enzyme mixture, 10 μL of water, and 4 μL of either the plasma miRNA or 250 nM of standard miRNA for 1 hour at 42°C, and 5 minutes at 95°C. The cDNA samples can be stored at −20°C.

Polymerase Chain Reaction

Multiple housekeeping genes are used in triplicate for data normalization and for analysis by the standard C_t method of quantification using StepOnePlus Real-Time PCR (Applied Biosystems, Foster City, CA). They also serve as controls for variability in sample loading. The sample testing is performed in equivalent with standards to evade batch effects as described next.

The miRNA standard cDNA is diluted in water. The standard curve is set up in triplicate with five points starting at 10,000, 5000, 2500, 1250, and 625 copy number. The plasma cDNA is diluted to 20 folds. The real time PCR reaction is set up with a total volume of 10 μL containing 5 μL of SYBR Green (Applied Biosystems); 1 μL of PCR primer mix; and 4 μL of either the diluted cDNA from miRNA standard or the plasma cDNA, using Standard Curve model. The plasma miRNA concentration is calculated in 10^{-2} pM units using the Quantity value *3.125/6.02/1000. The reproducibility of the qRT-PCR assay data confirms the efficient extraction of miRNAs from plasma samples.

The method described previously has no limitations or interferences with respect to miRNA extraction and RT-PCR.

METHODOLOGY USING THE MAIN RESOURCES OF FORMALIN-FIXED TISSUES

Because the availability of fresh or frozen tissue is typically limited, archival collections of formalin-fixed paraffin-embedded (FFPE) tissues are highly desirable and provide a rich source for the study of human disease. Tissue blocks are available worldwide from nearly every patient with well-documented clinical data including histopathologic reports, which makes it ideal to carry out research studies. The summarized methodology of plasma and fine-needle aspirates (FNA) samples is shown in **Fig. 2**. Of particular interest is that miRNA, because of its strong structure and smaller size, remains protected from degradation during fixation process, and requires only a small amount to perform miRNA expression profiles or RT-PCR. A recent study using clinical specimens from prostate cancer has demonstrated the use of this in the clinical context.[6] The following section highlights the collection of FNA from tumor mass and the fixation method.

FNA Tissue Collection

Diagnostic FNAs from tumor mass can be collected using 20–23 gauge needle from patients with pancreatic cancer (or other cancers) that underwent computerized

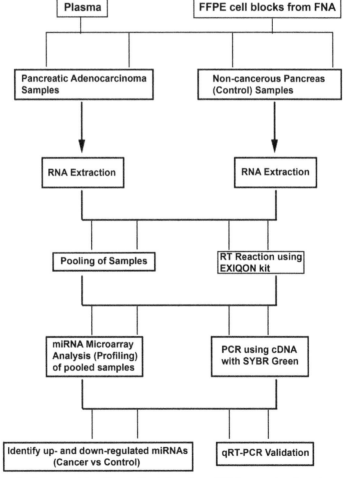

Fig. 2. Flow chart summarizing the methodology for miRNA research using plasma and FFPE cell blocks of FNA samples.

tomography or endoscopic ultrasound–guided biopsy. Diagnostic smears are stained using Diff-Quick staining (Mercedes Medical, Sarasota, FL). The aspirates are put in fixative fluid, centrifuged, and embedded in paraffin using standard protocol, and are stained by hematoxylin and eosin staining for the presence of tumor cells. Approximately 50 cells are required to obtain good quality and quantity of total RNA (consisting of miRNA) to perform quantitative RT-PCR (qRT-PCR). For the comparative purpose, normal pancreatic tissue that are further away from the pancreatic tumor (typically obtained from surgical specimens) can also be similarly fixed to serve as controls.

RNA Isolation

The miRNA is isolated from FFPE tissue using RNeasy Kit (QIAGEN, Valencia, CA) following manufacturer's protocol with a few modifications, which are described next. Four 10-μm thick and approximately 1 cm in diameter tissue curls are placed in 1 mL of xylene, mixed, and centrifuged for 2 minutes at room temperature. One milliliter of ethanol is added to the pellet and centrifuged for 2 minutes, and mixed with 240 μL of Buffer PKD along with 10 μL of proteinase K and incubated at 55°C, and then at 80°C for 15 minutes each. The mixture is then centrifuged, and the collected flow-through is mixed with 500 μL of buffer RBC to adjust binding conditions. The solution is mixed with ethanol and applied to the RNeasy column, and washed with buffer solution. The total RNA containing miRNA is eluted with RNase-free water. The purity of RNA is measured by the absorption ratio at 260/280 nm and quantified using Nano-Drop 2000 (Thermo Scientific, Pittsburgh, PA). The ratio of 260/280 typically ranges between 1.8 and 2.1.

Real-Time RT-PCR

The RT reaction is performed with SYBR Green miRNA-based assay using Exiqon-Universal cDNA synthesis kit (Exiqon). The RT reaction is set up with 10 μL of sample containing 2 μL of 5× RT buffer, 1 μL of enzyme mixture, 2 μL of water, and 10 ng of total RNA in 5 μL for 1 hour at 42°C and 5 minutes at 95°C. All reactions for PCR are carried out in triplicate using StepOnePlus Real-Time PCR (Applied Biosystems). The expression level of miRNAs is analyzed using C_t method.

MiRNA Profiling

The prognosis of patients with cancer remains poor. Hence, new biomarkers are essential for early detection of cancer progression. The miRNA profiling can be useful as biomarkers for differentiating tumor from normal samples either from plasma, FNA, or surgical tissue samples as discussed in many recent reports.[6,12,29,38,53] For example, equal amount of RNA containing miRNA and combined separately from control and patient samples can be analyzed for miRNA microarray profiling (LC Sciences, Houston, TX). The data are normalized using multiple housekeeping genes. Differentially regulated miRNAs between normal and cancer samples are analyzed using various statistical methodologies (eg, hierarchical clustering). Network analyses are accomplished using World Wide Web–based bioinformatics software programs, such as Ingenuity Pathway Analysis software (Ingenuity Systems, Redwood City, CA) functional network analysis. Pathway analysis is a new innovative tool that reveals the expression of deregulated[12] miRNAs and their putative targets in a signaling pathway.[6,54] Because each miRNA may have more than one target, miRNA-based therapy can be beneficial to target multiple signaling pathways, which include inhibition of oncogenic miRNAs by antisense oligonucleotides or by overexpression of tumor suppressor miRNA by precursor miRNAs.[6,30,44]

ADVANCES MADE IN CHARACTERIZING MIRNA PROFILING

Because there is an urgent need to investigate potential biomarkers for early detection of malignancies in a fast and simple way, miRNA research has made a significant impact on many types of cancer research, revealing basic gene expression changes toward identifying major signaling pathways involved in biomedical research. It empowers efficient profiling of deregulated miRNAs in plasma, serum, FFPE, and many other sample types because of their stability, which enables their detection and analysis thus leading to a potentially reliable biomarker. Profiling of miRNAs not only provides access to hundreds of expressed miRNAs in the sample, but also differentiates between healthy and diseased state. Some of the miRNAs are substantially upregulated or downregulated in cancer cells or tumor tissues relative to normal cells or normal tissues, permitting the identification of miRNA signature. Differential expression of lead candidate miRNAs can be individually further validated by RT-PCR. However, it is unlikely that any one of the conventional housekeeping genes will be sufficient to normalize the data. Hence, the use of multiple housekeeping genes for data normalization using the standard method of quantification may be the ideal way of performing miRNA profiling. Overall miRNA profiling is one of the most current methods to differentiate abnormally expressed miRNAs in a set of samples.

DIAGNOSTIC AND PROGNOSTIC IMPLICATIONS OF MIRNAS

Biomarkers that are predictive, prognostic, and diagnostic can be a valuable tool to clinicians in making important decisions about patient care.[6] The discovery of circulating miRNAs in plasma and serum, because of its noninvasive nature, are excellent biomarkers for a variety of cancer detection and prognostic purposes. We have previously shown circulating miRNAs as biomarkers in pancreatic cancer. A previous report by Ali and colleagues has identified a group of seven miRNAs including two oncogenic and five tumor suppressor miRNAs that were recognized and validated as a diagnostic marker in 50 plasma samples from patients with pancreatic cancer in comparison with healthy normal control subjects.[29] Similar reports on FNA from FFPE cell blocks in patients with pancreatic cancer also identified seven miRNAs that were differentially expressed in tumor cells compared with normal tissues.[12] These seven miRNAs both from plasma and FNA showed substantial differences in their expression level and hence may serve as diagnostic biomarkers in the detection of cancer. In addition, the Ingenuity networking pathway analysis in FNA study provided a unique strategy to study various signaling pathways, which revealed 15 biofunctional network groups relating to cancer, genetic disorder, and gastrointestinal disease that are expected to improve prognosis and response to certain therapies.[12] Other investigators also performed miRNA profiling in various other solid tumors to discover differentially expressed panel of miRNAs in pooled samples that reached excellent diagnostic properties to classify them as biomarker for cancer detection.[34,38,53,55] Novel high throughput multiplex technologies hold immense promise in this regard. However, before these can be clinically applicable, these need to be correlated with the morphologic and clinical findings to decipher those that are clinically relevant. Additional studies are needed to edify miRNA biomarkers to reduce patient mortality, morbidity, and introduce early diagnosis thereby reducing health care costs and applying these approaches to patient care.

SUMMARY

The miRNAs have immense potential in the clinical arena because they can be detected in the blood; serum; tissues (fresh and formalin-fixed paraffin embedded); and FNA specimens. Identification of novel molecular miRNAs and their target oncogenomic signatures has the potential to significantly impact clinical management. The discovery of miRNAs and their expression profile in a wide variety of cancers has led investigators to understand the key role of miRNAs as biomarkers during cancer progression. Incorporating miRNA expression profiling on tissue samples in the future may not only confirm diagnosis categorizing diseases and their subtypes but also may predict drug response in helping clinicians define the precise therapy to each individual. Moreover, increasing the knowledge of disease progression and tumor recurrence might also improve the development of personalized therapies. The most attractive feature of miRNA-based therapy is that a single miRNA could be useful for targeting multiple genes that are deregulated in cancers, which can be further investigated through systems biology and network analysis that allows designing cancer-specific personalized therapy. In summary, miRNAs are poised to provide diagnostic and prognostic markers for disease. However, miRNA-based therapy in human patients awaits clinical trials that will affirm miRNA application and open new areas of personalized medicine.

REFERENCES

1. Lei Z, Tan IB, Das K, et al. Identification of molecular subtypes of gastric cancer with different responses to PI3-kinase inhibitors and 5-fluorouracil. Gastroenterology 2013;145:554–65.
2. Elghannam DM, Ibrahim L, Ebrahim MA, et al. Association of MDR1 gene polymorphism (G2677T) with imatinib response in Egyptian chronic myeloid leukemia patients. Hematology 2013. [Epub ahead of print].
3. Tan J, Yu Q. Molecular mechanisms of tumor resistance to PI3K-mTOR targeted cancer therapy. Chin J Cancer 2013;32(7):376–9.
4. Lv X, Ma X, Hu Y. Furthering the design and the discovery of small molecule ATP-competitive mTOR inhibitors as an effective cancer treatment. Expert Opin Drug Discov 2013;8(8):991–1012.
5. Rai G, Vyjayanti VN, Dorjsuren D, et al. Small molecule inhibitors of the human apurinic/apyrimidinic endonuclease 1 (APE1). 2010.
6. Sethi S, Kong D, Land S, et al. Comprehensive molecular oncogenomic profiling and miRNA analysis of prostate cancer. Am J Transl Res 2013;5:200–11.
7. Sethi S, Sarkar FH. Evolving concept of cancer stem cells: role of micro-RNAs and their implications in tumor aggressiveness. J Carcinogene Mutagene 2011;(S1):005. http://dx.doi.org/10.4172/2157-2518.S1-005.
8. Hassan O, Ahmad A, Sethi S, et al. Recent updates on the role of microRNAs in prostate cancer. J Hematol Oncol 2012;5:9.
9. Bao L, Yan Y, Xu C, et al. MicroRNA-21 suppresses PTEN and hSulf-1 expression and promotes hepatocellular carcinoma progression through AKT/ERK pathways. Cancer Lett 2013;337(2):226–36.
10. Lei H, Zou D, Li Z, et al. MicroRNA-219-2-3p functions as a tumor suppressor in gastric cancer and is regulated by DNA methylation. PLoS One 2013;8:e60369.
11. Shen SN, Wang LF, Jia YF, et al. Upregulation of microRNA-224 is associated with aggressive progression and poor prognosis in human cervical cancer. Diagn Pathol 2013;8:69.
12. Ali S, Saleh H, Sethi S, et al. MicroRNA profiling of diagnostic needle aspirates from patients with pancreatic cancer. Br J Cancer 2012;107:1354–60.
13. Qazi AM, Gruzdyn O, Semaan A, et al. Restoration of E-cadherin expression in pancreatic ductal adenocarcinoma treated with microRNA-101. Surgery 2012;152:704–11.

14. Ahmad A, Sarkar SH, Bitar B, et al. Garcinol regulates EMT and Wnt signaling pathways in vitro and in vivo, leading to anticancer activity against breast cancer cells. Mol Cancer Ther 2012;11:2193–201.

15. Kong D, Heath E, Chen W, et al. Loss of let-7 up-regulates EZH2 in prostate cancer consistent with the acquisition of cancer stem cell signatures that are attenuated by BR-DIM. PLoS One 2012;7:e33729.

16. Ahmad A, Aboukameel A, Kong D, et al. Phosphoglucose isomerase/autocrine motility factor mediates epithelial-mesenchymal transition regulated by miR-200 in breast cancer cells. Cancer Res 2011;71:3400–9.

17. Kong D, Banerjee S, Ahmad A, et al. Epithelial to mesenchymal transition is mechanistically linked with stem cell signatures in prostate cancer cells. PLoS One 2010;5:e12445.

18. Baraniskin A, Kuhnhenn J, Schlegel U, et al. MicroRNAs in cerebrospinal fluid as biomarker for disease course monitoring in primary central nervous system lymphoma. J Neurooncol 2012;109:239–44.

19. Brunet VA, Pericay C, Moya I, et al. microRNA expression profile in stage III colorectal cancer: circulating miR-18a and miR-29a as promising biomarkers. Oncol Rep 2013;30:320–6.

20. Ulivi P, Foschi G, Mengozzi M, et al. Peripheral blood miR-328 expression as a potential biomarker for the early diagnosis of NSCLC. Int J Mol Sci 2013;14:10332–42.

21. Bi S, Cui Y, Li L. Dumbbell probe-mediated cascade isothermal amplification: a novel strategy for label-free detection of microRNAs and its application to real sample assay. Anal Chim Acta 2013;760:69–74.

22. Gu LQ, Wanunu M, Wang MX, et al. Detection of miRNAs with a nanopore single-molecule counter. Expert Rev Mol Diagn 2012;12:573–84.

23. Guan DG, Liao JY, Qu ZH, et al. mirExplorer: detecting microRNAs from genome and next generation sequencing data using the AdaBoost method with transition probability matrix and combined features. RNA Biol 2011;8:922–34.

24. Luo S. MicroRNA expression analysis using the Illumina microRNA-Seq Platform. Methods Mol Biol 2012;822:183–8.

25. Acunzo M, Romano G, Palmieri D, et al. Cross-talk between MET and EGFR in non-small cell lung cancer involves miR-27a and Sprouty2. Proc Natl Acad Sci U S A 2013;110:8573–8.

26. Yang J, Zhang W. New molecular insights into osteosarcoma targeted therapy. Curr Opin Oncol 2013;25:398–406.

27. Noguchi S, Iwasaki J, Kumazaki M, et al. Chemically modified synthetic microRNA-205 inhibits the growth of melanoma cells in vitro and in vivo. Mol Ther 2013;21:1204–11.

28. Dang Y, Luo D, Rong M, et al. Underexpression of miR-34a in hepatocellular carcinoma and its contribution towards enhancement of proliferating inhibitory effects of agents targeting c-MET. PLoS One 2013;8:e61054.

29. Ali S, Almhanna K, Chen W, et al. Differentially expressed miRNAs in the plasma may provide a molecular signature for aggressive pancreatic cancer. Am J Transl Res 2010;3:28–47.

30. Ali S, Banerjee S, Logna F, et al. Inactivation of Ink4a/Arf leads to deregulated expression of miRNAs in K-Ras transgenic mouse model of pancreatic cancer. J Cell Physiol 2012;227:3373–80.

31. Ali S, Ahmad A, Banerjee S, et al. Gemcitabine sensitivity can be induced in pancreatic cancer cells through modulation of miR-200 and miR-21 expression by curcumin or its analogue CDF. Cancer Res 2010;70:3606–17.

32. Liang Y, Ridzon D, Wong L, et al. Characterization of microRNA expression profiles in normal human tissues. BMC Genomics 2007;8:166.
33. Griffiths-Jones S. miRBase: microRNA sequences and annotation. Curr Protoc Bioinformatics 2010;29:12.9.1–12.9.10.
34. Gall TM, Frampton AE, Krell J, et al. Blood-based miRNAs as noninvasive diagnostic and surrogative biomarkers in colorectal cancer. Expert Rev Mol Diagn 2013;13:141–5.
35. Hermansen SK, Dahlrot RH, Nielsen BS, et al. MiR-21 expression in the tumor cell compartment holds unfavorable prognostic value in gliomas. J Neurooncol 2013; 111:71–81.
36. Si H, Sun X, Chen Y, et al. Circulating microRNA-92a and microRNA-21 as novel minimally invasive biomarkers for primary breast cancer. J Cancer Res Clin Oncol 2013;139:223–9.
37. Sicard F, Gayral M, Lulka H, et al. Targeting miR-21 for the therapy of pancreatic cancer. Mol Ther 2013;21(5):986–94.
38. Tang D, Shen Y, Wang M, et al. Identification of plasma microRNAs as novel noninvasive biomarkers for early detection of lung cancer. Eur J Cancer Prev 2013. [Epub ahead of print].
39. Yang SM, Huang C, Li XF, et al. miR-21 confers cisplatin resistance in gastric cancer cells by regulating PTEN. Toxicology 2013;306:162–8.
40. Liu R, Liao J, Yang M, et al. Circulating miR-155 expression in plasma: a potential biomarker for early diagnosis of esophageal cancer in humans. J Toxicol Environ Health A 2012;75:1154–62.
41. Yang M, Shen H, Qiu C, et al. High expression of miR-21 and miR-155 predicts recurrence and unfavourable survival in non-small cell lung cancer. Eur J Cancer 2013;49:604–15.
42. Zhang Y, Roccaro AM, Rombaoa C, et al. LNA-mediated anti-miR-155 silencing in low-grade B-cell lymphomas. Blood 2012;120:1678–86.
43. Yabushita S, Fukamachi K, Tanaka H, et al. Circulating microRNAs in serum of human K-ras oncogene transgenic rats with pancreatic ductal adenocarcinomas. Pancreas 2012;41:1013–8.
44. Ali S, Ahmad A, Aboukameel A, et al. Increased Ras GTPase activity is regulated by miRNAs that can be attenuated by CDF treatment in pancreatic cancer cells. Cancer Lett 2012;319:173–81.
45. Bhutia YD, Hung SW, Krentz M, et al. Differential processing of let-7a precursors influences RRM2 expression and chemosensitivity in pancreatic cancer: role of LIN-28 and SET oncoprotein. PLoS One 2013;8:e53436.
46. Hu X, Guo J, Zheng L, et al. The heterochronic microRNA let-7 inhibits cell motility by regulating the genes in the actin cytoskeleton pathway in breast cancer. Mol Cancer Res 2013;11:240–50.
47. Kang HW, Crawford M, Fabbri M, et al. A mathematical model for microRNA in lung cancer. PLoS One 2013;8:e53663.
48. Zaman MS, Maher DM, Khan S, et al. Current status and implications of microRNAs in ovarian cancer diagnosis and therapy. J Ovarian Res 2012;5:44.
49. Jusufovic E, Rijavec M, Keser D, et al. let-7b and miR-126 are down-regulated in tumor tissue and correlate with microvessel density and survival outcomes in non–small–cell lung cancer. PLoS One 2012;7:e45577.
50. Xia XM, Jin WY, Shi RZ, et al. Clinical significance and the correlation of expression between Let-7 and K-ras in non-small cell lung cancer. Oncol Lett 2010;1:1045–7.
51. Vogt M, Munding J, Gruner M, et al. Frequent concomitant inactivation of miR-34a and miR-34b/c by CpG methylation in colorectal, pancreatic, mammary,

ovarian, urothelial, and renal cell carcinomas and soft tissue sarcomas. Virchows Arch 2011;458:313–22.

52. Krutzfeldt J, Rajewsky N, Braich R, et al. Silencing of microRNAs in vivo with 'antagomirs'. Nature 2005;438:685–9.

53. Callari M, Dugo M, Musella V, et al. Comparison of microarray platforms for measuring differential microRNA expression in paired normal/cancer colon tissues. PLoS One 2012;7:e45105.

54. Azmi AS, Ali S, Banerjee S, et al. Network modeling of CDF treated pancreatic cancer cells reveals a novel c-myc-p73 dependent apoptotic mechanism. Am J Transl Res 2011;3:374–82.

55. Lang MF, Yang S, Zhao C, et al. Genome-wide profiling identified a set of miRNAs that are differentially expressed in glioblastoma stem cells and normal neural stem cells. PLoS One 2012;7:e36248.

Diagnostic Molecular Microbiology: A 2013 Snapshot

Marilynn Ransom Fairfax, MD, PhD*, Hossein Salimnia, PhD

KEYWORDS

- Molecular microbiology • PCR • Probe tests
- Rapid molecular diagnosis of infections • Multiplex PCR panels • MALDI TOF
- Nuclear magnetic resonance

KEY POINTS

- In 2013, diagnostic molecular testing has a large and increasing role in the diagnosis of infectious diseases.
- It has evolved significantly since the first probe tests were FDA approved in the early 1990s.
- It has evolved beyond PCR or even RT-PCR to include highly multiplexed PCR carried out in microfluidic pouch systems, matrix-assisted laser desorption/ionization time of flight, and nuclear magnetic resonance.

INTRODUCTION

When Kary Mullis developed the polymerase chain reaction (PCR) in 1983, its potential benefits were obvious to clinical microbiologists: faster, cheaper, more accurate detection and enumeration of all organisms in a specimen, without waiting for culture. We also wanted simultaneous antimicrobial susceptibility testing. Our dreams are now coming true. Multiplex arrays are approved or in development for the diagnosis of respiratory and gastrointestinal infections direct from patient specimens within less than an hour. An array was FDA cleared in August, 2013, that can detect common bacterial and fungal agents of bloodstream infections, as well as several important antibiotic-resistant genes, within about an hour after the culture bottle turns positive. Microbiology lines are available, starting with automated plate streakers and ending with molecular identification of organisms grown on solid media. Humans must still view the culture plates, perhaps on a television screen, and select colonies to analyze.

"Cheaper" is an ambiguous target. Microbiology laboratories are diagnostic facilities that drive subsequent therapy. Increased laboratory costs for more rapid

Department of Pathology, Wayne State University School of Medicine, and Microbiology Division, Detroit Medical Center University Laboratories, 4201 Saint Antoine, Detroit, MI 48201, USA
* Corresponding author.
E-mail address: mfairfax@dmc.org

Clin Lab Med 33 (2013) 787–803
http://dx.doi.org/10.1016/j.cll.2013.08.003
labmed.theclinics.com
0272-2712/13/$ – see front matter © 2013 Elsevier Inc. All rights reserved.

microbial identification have been shown to result in earlier use of appropriate antibiotics, shorter lengths of hospital stay, and better outcomes, decreasing overall health care costs.[1–3] Diagnosis of persistent human papilloma virus infections followed by appropriate therapeutic interventions should reduce the incidence of cervical carcinomas, the cost of treatment, and the attributable morbidity and mortality.

New technologies have enabled microbiologic investigations that were not included in our original dreams. NextGen sequencing can detect and quantify populations of organisms in patient specimens. This raises the possibility of distinguishing pathogenic organisms, present in high numbers, from colonizers that are generally presumed to be present in lower numbers. Certain colonic organism profiles appear to correlate with the development of cardiovascular disease.[4] A patient's colonic flora could be analyzed, and if the profile were unfavorable, the bacteria could be eradicated and replaced.

Tests in use in 2013 have evolved significantly and will continue to do so. Thus, this article is a snapshot of rapidly changing diagnostic microbiology laboratory techniques. Because of space constraints, emphasis has been placed on tests with high market share in diagnostic microbiology and on those with technologies that are personally regarded by the authors as particularly interesting. The role of specimen processing in concentrating nucleic acid targets and removing inhibitors of amplification is largely neglected, despite its important role in the sensitivity of the assay. Most techniques mentioned here involve RT-PCR, unless otherwise specified. RT-PCR lowers the incidence of amplicon contamination in the laboratory, and has allowed many nucleic acid amplification techniques to come "out of the closet," but does not prevent specimen contamination. The authors have also attempted to select only one current citation to support most points, and these selections are arbitrary. Failure to mention a publication, technique, or trade name should not be construed as denigrating that article, technique, or manufacturer.

PROBE TECHNIQUES

The first molecular diagnostic tests approved by the Food and Drug Administration (FDA) were probe techniques. The probes were synthesized by molecular techniques, but the clinical laboratory performed only hybridization and detection. Many probe tests are still in wide use today because they fill important niches. Some involve novel detection methodologies.

Hybridization-Protection Assays

Among the first FDA-approved molecular tests were the Gen-Probe ([San Diego, CA], which became a wholly owned subsidiary of Hologic [Bedford, MA] in 2012). Pace 2 probe hybridization protection techniques for the diagnosis of *Chlamydia trachomatis* (CT) and *Neisseria gonorrhoeae* (NG) from patient specimens. They have been largely been replaced by more sensitive amplification tests. A number of their AccuProbe culture confirmation tests remain available. Among them are *Mycobacterium tuberculosis* (TB) complex, *Mycobacterium avium, Mycobacterium intracellulare* (separately or together), *Mycobacterium kansasii, and Mycobacterium gordoni*. In addition, there are 3 tests for dimorphic fungi: *Histoplasma capsulatum* (which also detects *H capsulatum var. dubosi*), *Blastomyces dermatididis* (which also detects *Paracoccidioides brasiliensis*), and *Coccidioides immitis*. These and other tests available from the same manufacturer all use most of the same reagents and instrumentation, which facilitates the use of multiple assays in the same laboratory.

These tests succeed because they target ribosomal RNA (rRNA), which is present in up to 10^5 copies per organism. In bacterial ribosomes, there are common sequences, as well as genus-specific and species-specific sequences. The culture confirmation tests remain viable because they are intended to detect organisms in visible colonies or in liquid medium with detectable growth. Thus, 2 amplification steps have already been performed by nature. Sensitivities reported in the Hologic/Gen-Probe package inserts range from 98% to 100%.

At development, these assays were novel: they were nonradioactive and performed totally in solution, with 1 sample transfer step and no nucleic acid extraction. The hybridization-protection assays are based on the differential sensitivity of the acridinium ester, which is used to distinguish the relatively labile ester on nonhybridized probes from the more stable form in DNA-RNA hybrids. This detection system is also used in this manufacturer's nucleic acid amplification tests (NAATs). All the AccuProbe assays are similar but the nucleic acid release steps are variable, depending on the ease of disruption of the organism.

Many laboratories have used the mycobacterial probes for approximately 20 years, and have found no reason to argue with the FDA-approved sensitivity and specificity, both of which exceed 99.6%.[5] Although *Mycobacterium celatum* in high concentrations also reacts with the TB complex probe,[6] we have seen only 1 in 20 years (Fairfax, unpublished data, 2013).

The mycobacterial probe tests are particularly valuable when used in conjunction with liquid medium or 7H11 thin-plate techniques[7] used for the rapid detection and identification of mycobacteria required by the College of American Pathologists (Northfield, IL). Thin-plate colonies can be probed the day they are detected, and their morphology can be used as a guide to selection of the appropriate probe. This represents significant time and money saving, although it does not eliminate the need to grow *M tuberculosis* for susceptibility testing. If there is only one visible colony and if the probe result is negative, whether due to inadequate sample, improper probe selection, or growth of an organism not recognized by the probe, one must wait for the colony to regrow before further analysis (Fairfax and Salimnia, unpublished data). Cultures in Middlebrook 7H9 broth must be AFB stained to confirm the presence of mycobacteria[8] and then probed with all 4 probes.

Hybrid Capture Technique

Since the 1940s, Pap smears have contributed to great advances in the prevention and diagnosis of cervical carcinoma. In the 1980s and 1990s, it was recognized that infection with human papilloma virus (HPV) is necessary but not sufficient for the development of cervical carcinoma. More than 100 HPV genotypes exist, of which 13 are associated with a high risk of cervical carcinoma (16, 18, 31, 33, 35, 39, 45, 51, 52, 56, 58, 59, 68). More than 70% of sexually active women become infected with HPV. Most infections, even with high-risk organisms, resolve without apparent sequellae. Why others progress is still unknown.[9] The Digene Hybrid Capture 2 (hc2; Qiagen, Gaithersburg, MD) is FDA approved for primary screening, and to determine whether women with atypical squamous cells of undetermined significance should be subjected to culposcopy. It may be used with the Cytyc PreservCyt Solution for the Cytyc ThinPrep Pap Test (Hologic).[10]

In the first step, the patient specimen is allowed to react with a pool of RNA probes designed to hybridize specifically to the DNA of high-risk HPV strains. Antibody to RNA/DNA hybrids coats the wells of a microtiter plate and captures any hybrids. After washing away unbound specimen and reagents, detector antihybrid antibodies, each conjugated with multiple molecules of alkaline phosphatase, bind to each captured target, amplifying the signal. A colorless substrate for the alkaline phosphatase is added and chemiluminescence develops proportional to the amount of second antibody bound.

More sensitive tests, typically involving target amplification, have been devised, but most clinical outcomes data are available with hc2. The need for more sensitivity has been questioned, as hc2 has already been shown to be sensitive, but not highly specific, for the development of cervical intraepithelial neoplasia or overt malignancy. The presence of high-risk DNA below the detection limit of hc2 appears to be associated with a low risk for malignancy.[9] However, new information suggests that infections acquired in the early years of sexual activity may reactivate with aging.[11] If this is supported by further studies, more sensitive assays might be indicated. There is also a suggestion that unusual HPV strains may cause cervical carcinoma or precursor lesions in restricted populations.[12] Thus, the strains included in the assay may need periodic review.

bDNA

Several generations of the Versant branched-chain (b) DNA signal amplification viral load tests (Bayer Corp, Berkeley, CA) have been used for determination of cytomegalovirus (CMV), HIV, and hepatitis B virus (HBV) viral loads for 15 to 20 years. The most recent bDNA HIV viral load assay is version 3.0, and the current lower limit of quantification (LLQ) is approximately 8 to 10 nucleic acid targets per reaction, or about 73 copies/mL,[13] in contrast to the LLQ of 10 copies/mL for the latest nucleic acid amplification viral load techniques (see later in this article). Although overnight incubation has been standard, a new algorithm that can be performed in 9 hours has been published.[14]

The bDNA technique resembles a "molecular tree" (**Fig. 1**). The wells of microtiter plates are coated with capture probes, which bind the target extender, then the target. Three more hybridization steps occur, with significant amplification at each. In the last, multiple alkaline phosphatase-coupled probes bind to the branched amplifier probes. Each enzyme converts multiple molecules of its colorless substrate into colored end product, allowing the detection of small numbers of initial targets.

bDNA is unaffected by amplicon contamination (because there are no amplicons) and relatively insensitive to inhibitors that plague many NAATs. It is also less sensitive to problems resulting from freezing specimens in plasma preparation (PP) tubes.[15] This mode of specimen transport is no longer recommended for amplification-based viral load determinations, as DNA escaping from the gel matrix in the PP tube can increase the apparent viral load by hundreds of copies/mL, which was unnoticeable when the viral loads were routinely in the thousands or tens of thousands,[15] but which is unacceptable today, when viral loads of <20 are frequently reported (see later in this article).

substrate

plate – capture probe -- capture extender – target – target extender – preamplifier – amplifier – alk phos probe ↓

product

Fig. 1. The bDNA "molecular tree" technique.

Peptide Nucleic Acid Fluorescence In Situ Hybridization

Peptide nucleic acid fluorescence in situ hybridization (PNA-FISH) (AdvanDx, Inc, Woburn, MA) has accelerated the diagnosis of sepsis. Common agents of sepsis can be identified in about an hour after the blood culture bottle has been Gram stained. Although behaving like a standard FISH assay, the PNA-FISH probes consist of an uncharged peptide backbone to which the bases are attached. This is thought to allow the probes to enter the permeablized bacterial cell more easily and then bind more tightly to the negatively charged rRNA target. Numerous publications confirm that use of this technique for rapid identification of the common organisms growing in the blood culture bottles improves antibiotic stewardship and shortens length of stay.[1,2] Depending on the patient, identification of a coagulase-negative *Staphylococcus* may facilitate discontinuation of antibiotics and early discharge (Salimnia and Fairfax, unpublished results, 2013).

Our high-throughput laboratory (>200 blood cultures per day) was an early adapter of the staphylococcal, enterococcal, and candida probes, although we do not currently use those for gram-negative organisms because we determined that the test's ability to identify only 2 or 3 organisms was not cost effective for our complex patient population. We run the gram positive and fungal assays once per shift. In general, the identifications are congruent with culture and identification on the MicroScan (WalkAway 96si; Siemans HealthCare Diagnostics, West Sacramento, CA). Rare misses have occurred in mixed infections due to failure to detect very low numbers of *Staphylococcus aureus* against the background of a much higher number of coagulase-negative *Staphylococcus*, or similar low numbers of *Enterococcus faecalis* in a background of other *Enterococcus* spp. On review of the slides, the previously undetected organism was seen (Salimnia, unpublished results). This no longer occurs as our technologists are alert to this possibility. In a few, rare situations, the PNA-FISH and the MicroScan have disagreed. These discordant results have been resolved in favor of PNA-FISH by 16S rRNA sequencing.[16] Depending on how one resolves the results of the mixed cultures described previously, the sensitivity and specificity of PNA-FISH in our laboratory approximate 100%.

Red/green fluorescent probe kits at this time include coagulase-negative *Staphylococcus* (green) versus *S aureus* (red), *Enterococcus* sp (red) versus *E* faecalis (green), *Escherichia coli* (green) versus *Pseudomonas aerugenosa* (red), and *Candida albicans* (green) versus *Candida glabrata* (red). Two tests use 3-color (red, yellow, green; traffic light) fluorescence: gram-negative rods (*E coli* [green], *Klebsiella pneumoniae* [yellow], and *P aerugenosa* [red]) and Candida. In the *Candida* assay, *C albicans* and *Candida parapsilosis*, both susceptible to most antifungals, fluoresce green, *Candida tropicalis* fluoresces yellow, and both *C glabrata* and *Candida krusei* fluoresce red. Also approved are 20-minute, 2-color tests for *Staphylococcus* sp versus *S aureus* and *Enterococcus* sp versus *E faecalis*, potentially allowing the reporting of a preliminary identification at the same time as the Gram stain. A universal bacterial probe is available as an analyte-specific reagent (ASR), as are specific probes for *Acinetobacter, Candida dublinensis*, and *C parapsilosis* (AdvanDx Web Products section of site, queried September 5, 2013).

Affirm VPIII Microbial Identification Test

The VPIII probe test (Becton Dickinson [BD], Franklin Lakes, NJ) is intended for the diagnosis of vaginitis/vaginosis, conditions causing millions of physician visits annually. It detects rRNA from *Gardnerella vaginalis*, used as an indicator for bacterial vaginosis (BV), *C albicans*, and *Trichomonas vaginalis*. The sensitivity has been adjusted to avoid giving positive results with low concentrations of *G vaginalis* and *C albicans,* which often colonize the normal vagina. It is formatted to be performed in a cassette superficially resembling the lateral flow tests used for the serologic detection of influenza or rotavirus antigens and was the first FDA-approved molecular test based on lateral flow. After collection on a proprietary swab, the specimen is lysed to release the nucleic acids, buffered to stabilize the nucleic acids and establish stringency, and added to the cassette, which is incubated at the proper temperature for nucleic acid hybridization. The cassette contains 5 "beads," each coupled to a capture probe: 1 for each of the 3 analytes, plus positive and negative controls. Next, enzyme-linked detector probes bind to specific sequences on the target organism's rRNA. Unbound sample components and probes are washed away. A colorless substrate is converted to a blue product if sufficient target and detector probe have bound. A blue "bead" indicates a positive result.[17]

Numerous publications have revealed that health care providers are significantly less accurate than VPIII for the diagnosis of significant candidiasis, and T vaginalis. The role of the VPIII in the diagnosis of BV is still the subject of some debate, as G vaginalis is found both in the presence and the absence of BV. In an analysis of results from our laboratory, mixed infections were common. Of those patients positive for T vaginalis, almost 2/3 were positive for one or both of the other organisms.[18] FDA-approved NAATs with higher sensitivity and a higher price are also available for T vaginalis (Hologic/Gen-Probe).[19]

QUALITATIVE NAATS

This section concentrates on tests that give a positive or negative result for 1, 2, or 3 analytes. Highly multiplexed NAATs are discussed in a section entitled "Highly Multiplexed PCR Panels."

Sexually Transmitted Disease Testing

Culture, immunoassay, and probe tests for both NG and CT are less sensitive than NAATs, and NAATs have been the standard of care since the late 1990s, although certain jurisdictions require culture for legal cases. Despite the relatively long history of NAAT use, the testing modalities are still undergoing significant changes that are mentioned later in this article. It should be noted that, because of updates in targets and instrumentation, previously published comparisons may no longer apply.

Although NAAT is generally assumed to mean PCR, this is not always the case: when PCR was patent protected, other innovative amplification techniques were developed. Two of these are isothermal, avoiding the requirement for expensive thermal cyclers: strand-displacement amplification (SDA; BD Probe Tec ET and Q^x) and transcription-mediated amplification (TMA; Aptima Combo 2; Hologic Gen-Probe). These are both described in detail in the methods article. The TMA assay targets organism-specific rRNA sequences in each organism: 23S rRNA for CT and 16S rRNA for NG. It begins with target capture on magnetic beads, and ends with the hybridization protection assay similar to those previously described for the AccuProbe tests, although each species of detector probe is attached to a different acrydinium ester. One flashes very rapidly and its chemiluminescence attenuates before the other begins to fluoresce (glow). Thus, they can be detected sequentially in the same tube.[20]

The BD SDA CT assay targets an open reading frame in the cryptic CT plasmid.[21] The testing is very complicated to describe (see the methods article), but much simpler to perform, especially on automated instrumentation. The manufacturers of both isothermal amplification tests sell high-throughput analyzers using the same (or modified, as in SDA Q^x) technology. Two PCR-based tests, by Roche (Roche Cobas Amplicor [RCA]; Roche Molecular Diagnostics, Pleasonton, CA) and Abbott (Abbott RealTime [ART]; Abbott Molecular, Des Plaines, IL) CT/NG assay (on their m2000 automated platform) are also major players in the huge market for diagnosis of CT and NG. Both PCR-based CT tests originally targeted sequences in the cryptic plasmid.[22]

The older tests are FDA approved for cervical swabs, genital swabs, and urine. Several are approved for physician-collected or self-collected vaginal swabs. Both TMA and SDA are approved for use with the specimen collected for the Thin Prep PAP smear technique,[20,23] although the newer versions may not yet be approved for all specimen types. To prevent contamination, the sample for nucleic acid amplification must be removed before processing the cytology sample for cellular analysis.[20,23] The specificities of all the assays are comparable, although the RCA has been reported to detect nongonorrhoeae *Neisseria*,[24,25] and their sensitivities appear to be adequate for genital specimens, with TMA appearing slightly more sensitive than standard SDA, both of which may be slightly better than either PCR assay.[21,22,24,26] In general, the sensitivities of all 4 tests are lower for CT than for NG, perhaps due to a lower organism burden for CT.[22]

The high-throughput, automated BD SDA assays for NG and CT (ProbeTec Q[x]) performed in extracted mode on their Viper System have improved sensitivity. This may be due partly to target changes and in part to contaminants being removed by use of a magnetic, ferric oxide bead-capture system. The ferric oxide technique could be generalizable because it does not require the presence of specific target sequences. Briefly, the bacteria are lysed in a high-pH solution. The pH is lowered to generate a positive charge on the ferric oxide particles, which bind the negatively charged nucleic acids. The particles are magnetically captured and washed, and the bound DNA is eluted by raising the pH. The extracted DNA is buffered to a pH appropriate for the amplification assay.[21,23]

Recently, several studies have been performed to extend these tests to rectal and oropharyngeal specimens. Although not yet FDA approved for these sources, their sensitivities and specificities appear adequate with the exception of oropharyngeal NG by RCA.[24,25] The RCA test has been shown to detect nongonorrhoeal *Neisseriaceae* and is not appropriate for nongenital testing.[24,25] Perhaps in response to this, Roche has introduced a new version of its STD tests (Cobas 4800), which targets the DR-9 region of NG, improving its specificity and also has changes, described later in this article, that improve its ability to test for CT.[24] This is not yet approved in the United States.

How long we will be able to continue using these tests is unclear, because problems have arisen with both CT and NG. A CT strain with a 377-base pair (bp) deletion in the cryptic plasmid that includes the original targets of both PCR tests has been detected in Sweden, where in 2009 it comprised 24% to 45% of CT-positive specimens.[27,28] The organism is rare in the rest of Europe and has not been detected in the United States.[28] Roche and Abbott have both modified their assays to include a second target sequence: *omp1* for Roche and a second region of the cryptic plasmid for Abbott.[24]

NG resistance to each recommended drug regimen has occurred after wide use of that antibiotic; resistance to cefepime been detected and is becoming more prevalent in the United States.[29] Transportation kits for these molecular tests are not compatible with culture and susceptibility testing, which is also significantly less sensitive. Thus, it appears that further molecular analysis of specimens that test positive for NG may be required to detect antibiotic-resistant genes. Such tests are not commercially available. The sequences best included in such assays remain to be determined and probably will need to be changed with time.

Additional tests for other urogenital pathogens are being added to the testing formats. TMA testing for *T vaginalis* was recently FDA approved and is more sensitive than VPIII.[19] Testing for HSV 1 and 2 from swabs of external anogenital lesions is also available from BD in their Q[x] format.[30]

Other Qualitative Assays

Hologic-Gen-Probe manufactures several widely used qualitative, TMA-based microbiology tests; included among these are a direct test for *M tuberculosis* and the Procleix Ultrio Plus assay (Ultrio), which has also been licensed to Novartis (Emoryville, CA). This latter assay (without the Plus) has long been approved for detection of HIV and HCV in specimens from blood donors and from organ donors, both living and deceased, but is not intended for the diagnostic workup of the diseases in the general population. Testing a pool of samples from up to 16 blood donor units is approved for blood bank testing. Recently, the FDA approved the inclusion of HBV in this assay, and it has been renamed Ultrio Plus. It contains several HIV targets that allow it to detect HIV-1 (several strains) and HIV-2. Because test results are generally negative and high sensitivity is necessary, inclusion of an internal control is essential. This uses the "flash technology," while a positive result gives rise to a "glow" (see previously). Components of positive pools are retested individually and then by assays for each individual analyte.[31]

A recent article contains a listing of more than 135 published RT-PCR assays developed for detection of 32 species of bacteria.[32] This list does not include multiplexed tests or assays for viruses. The investigator acknowledged that the list is incomplete and commented that most are laboratory-developed tests, with only 35 (counted from his list) being commercially available, whether FDA approved or not. This emphasizes the need for more rapid commercial development and FDA-approval methods.

Although cyber green, a nonspecific detector, is still used occasionally, 3 main molecular detection systems are used: dual hybridization (fluorescent resonance energy transfer [FRET]), TaqMan, and molecular beacon. The FRET detector consists of 2 different probes, complementary to adjacent sequences on the target amplicon, and each attached to a different fluor. When activated by incident UV light, the first fluor emits energy at an unmonitored wavelength. If the second probe is bound adjacent to it, the energy is transferred to the second flour, which then emits light at the wavelength monitored by the sensor. At the end of the PCR assay, a melting curve for the amplicon-probe complex can be generated. The melting temperature (Tm) is characteristic of each amplicon-probe combination. If there is a mismatch between the probe and the amplicon, the melting temperature decreases.[33] The Tm difference has been exploited in a test that distinguishes between herpes simplex 1 and 2 (Roche). The PCR primers bind sequences common to both viruses within the HSV DNA polymerase gene. The amplicon detector probes match the HSV-2 sequence, which differs from that of HSV-1 by 2 bp. Melting curve analysis reveals a reproducible Tm for HSV-2 that is about 10°C higher than that exhibited by HSV-1.[34] Occasional mutant HSV strains have been detected that have intermediate melting temperatures. These can be reported as positive for HSV, but the type is not clear. Types 1 and 2 could be distinguished by sequencing the amplicons, by using an assay employing a different target sequence, or by the Tm of the amplicon, which is said to be 0.9°C higher for the HSV-2 variant than the type 1 variant.[35]

The MultiCode RTx system uses an unusual PCR amplification technique in which no detector probe is used and in which the fluorescence actually decreases as amplification progresses. It was developed by EraGen BioSciences, Inc (Madison, WI; acquired by Luminex Corporation [Austin, TX] in 2011). Their Multicode-RTx Herpes simplex virus 1 and 2 kit was FDA approved in 2011. MultiCode RTx assays use 2 unusual nucleotide bases iC (2-deoxy-5-methylisocytidine) and iG (2′-deoxy-isoguanoside) that base pair only to one another and that are efficiently incorporated into PCR products. iG is put at the 5′ end of the RTx primers with a fluor covalently linked nearby. The reaction mix contains iC covalently linked to a quencher. In the initial cycle amplification, the iG, with its attached fluor, appears at the 5′ end of the nascent amplicon strands. When these serve as templates for copying in the other direction, an iC, with its attached quencher is added to the 3′ end of the new strand, opposite the iG and its fluor. The approximation of fluor and quencher decreases the fluorescence. In melting curve analysis, fluorescence increases as the amplicons melt, and the Tm allows determination of the nature of the analyte.[36] Although these RT-PCR assays are qualitative, detection is based on the determination of a CT, as with any other standard RT-PCR. Comparison of CTs can be used to provide a rough quantification of the amount of target DNA.[37]

QUANTITATIVE TECHNIQUES

Because of space constraints, comments on quantitative PCR in clinical microbiology are confined mainly to NAATs used for HIV viral load testing, although there are also FDA-approved quantitative RT-PCR assays for HCV, HBV, and recently for CMV. The trend is to make the assays referable to a World Health Organization international standard. Quantitative techniques have advanced significantly since the early days when Alice Huang first demonstrated that quantitative PCR was possible (for a detailed discussion and review of the literature, see Fairfax and Salimnia[33]).

RT-PCR is inherently semiquantitative. Theoretically, one can construct a standard curve of copy number versus CT and determine the quantity of analyte in a patient specimen by referring to the curve. However, variations in extraction efficiency and the presence of inhibitors can introduce significant errors, particularly at low levels of analyte, when one is attempting to distinguishing "only a few" from "none." One relatively straightforward method to overcome this problem includes the addition of a control target or quantitation standard (QS) into the patient sample before extraction. The target and the QS are extracted, amplified, and detected together, controlling for the extraction and for any inhibitors present. The ideal QS should be the same size and base composition as the target to be quantified, with the same primer binding sites. It should differ enough in sequence that the detector probe or probes for the target do not bind to it, and its own detector probe should fluoresce at a different wavelength from that of the target. Then, quantitation should be a simple mathematical calculation.[33] However, at low target concentrations, the standard curve is no longer straight. Roche has incorporated complex mathematical calculations into its recent viral load assays to account for this divergence.

The statistics of small numbers impact the detection of fewer than 10 targets per reaction mix. What is called "digital PCR" exploits this. For each specimen, multiple reactions are conducted in such small volumes (emulsified droplets, for example) that some contain no targets, whereas others will contain only one or a few. From the volume of sample in each reaction droplet, the number of positive and negative reactions, and the Poisson distribution, one can calculate the number of targets in the original sample. No FDA-approved assays are yet based on this intriguing technique.

Conversations have recently begun about possible "cures" of HIV infection, and as highly active antiretroviral therapy and improved plasma HIV viral load techniques converge, discussions have ensued about how to evaluate residual virus in well-controlled or possibly cured individuals. The most sensitive assays for determination of low-level infection are likely to be assays for HIV DNA copies in single cells. How to determine which ones are replication-competent is crucial to this discussion. Aside from circulating CD4 cells, what cells should be investigated is unclear at this time. This active area of investigation was recently reviewed by Strain and Richman,[38] who discussed very low level contamination, signal-to-noise ratios in PCR testing, single-cell PCR, and other techniques that are beyond the scope of this article.

With respect to HIV quantification in plasma, further considerations affect testing and result interpretation. The most obvious problem results from the increase in sensitivity as the assays improve. Patients who were told that their virus levels were "undetectable," suddenly have quantifiable virus. Time-consuming correlations between viral load and prognosis have to be redone for each new, more sensitive assay. Sequence differences between the numerous organism strains and the inherent mutability of the organisms also make accurate quantification difficult, especially for RNA viruses, such as HIV and HCV. One must target a stable sequence. However, the viral RNA polymerase enzymes are error prone and lack proofreading activity. Changes in the genetic sequence, particularly in the primer or probe-binding sites, may reduce detected viral load. Minority quasi-species also cause problems (see later in this article). It appears that more than one target will be necessary for future assays.

Because approval and release of diagnostic tests by different manufacturers are not coordinated, it is difficult to find articles comparing the performance of the latest offerings by different companies. Two current assays for HIV quantification in the United States are the Roche Cobas AmpliPrep Cobas TaqMan HIV viral load version 2.0 (CAP/CTM2) and the Abbott RealTime HIV-1 assay (ART HIV). The 2 assays have different lower limits of quantitation (LLQs), 20 c/mL for CAP/CTM2 and 40 c/mL for ART HIV, which introduces difficulties in comparison. They have, however, been compared in 2 recent articles.[39,40] Sire and colleagues[39] extrapolated the ART HIV curves, and found that 10 of 17 specimens that were quantifiable by the CAP/CTM2 but not by the ART HIV could actually be quantified. The assays correlated well ($r = 0.96$[38]), although CAP/CTM2 was more than 0.5 $\log_{10}$ higher than the ART HIV in 20% of 51 samples, whereas the ART HIV was more than 0.5 $\log_{10}$ higher in only 2 of them.[39] Whose result is more accurate remains to be determined.

HIGHLY MULTIPLEXED PCR PANELS

This section focuses only on highly multiplexed assays, roughly defined as those detecting more than 10 targets. Although many assays for individual etiology agents of disease are available, testing for individual organisms is often uninformative. Numerous viral and some bacterial agents of respiratory disease cause similar symptoms. It is usually not obvious which agent or agents are infecting a given patient. Even at the peak of an influenza epidemic, an individual may be infected with respiratory syncytial virus instead or concurrently. Furthermore, mixed infections are more common than many had imagined.[41,42] Some virus infections are treatable, and others have different isolation requirements if the patient is hospitalized.[42] Thus, molecular panels that could detect multiple etiologic agents of diseases clearly are desirable. Four multiplex respiratory panels are FDA approved at this writing: Luminex xTAG RVP (xRVP) and RVP Fast (xRVPF) (Luminex Diagnostics, Toronto, Canada); Film Array Respiratory Panel (FARP; BioFire Diagnostics [formerly Idaho Technologies], Salt Lake City, UT), and eSensor Respiratory Panel (eSRP) (GenMark Diagnostics, Carlsbad, CA). The FARP has the most targets, including 3 bacteria. One head-to-head comparison of all 4 test modalities was recently published.[43] The various analytes differ in sensitivity and specificity, but this study found that the eSRP had 100% sensitivity for all analytes compared. The xRVP was second, and more sensitive than the xRVPF, which was similar to the FARP. These results will require confirmation by other researchers, as Babady and colleagues[41] found the FARP to be more sensitive than the xRVPFfor many analytes. All tests are capable of detecting mixed infections.

Ultimately the final decision as to which test to implement in one's laboratory may come down to questions of cost, hands-on time, complexity, and convenience. The FARP provides a result within about 1 hour, requiring only minutes of hands-on time, but can handle only 1 sample at a time. It seems ideally suited to a medium-sized laboratory where technologists without specialized molecular expertise can perform the tests. Some larger laboratories have bought multiple instruments to facilitate throughput. But surge capacity may be lacking. The others are batch instruments, but they require sample extraction before testing, and amplicon manipulation afterward, which may confine them to a "PCR laboratory." Each handles 21 samples per run. None is suitable for 2 runs per shift, although staggered technologist start times could allow it with the xRVPF. The xRVP and eSRP require 7 to 8 hours for results.[43]

A problem with panels is that they tend to maximize the number of analytes detected in their initial offering, based on instrument constraints. Adding something new seems to require that something old be removed. FDA reapproval requires significant financial outlays for any change, and new respiratory viruses keep appearing. Newly detected viruses since 2001 include human metapneumoviruses (2001), severe acute respiratory syndrome (SARS; 2003), human bocavirus (2005), new influenza A viruses (H1N1, 2009; H7N9, 2013), and now, Middle East respiratory syndrome corona virus (MERS-CoV; 2012), the latter 2 of which apparently have not (yet) appeared in the United States but apparently have a high mortality rate.[44–46] The human metapneumoviruses and human bocavirus are included in some of the previously mentioned assays. It is not clear whether MERS-CoV can be detected by the coronavirus detector systems in these assays, but if so, it could not be distinguished from those that cause more common respiratory infections. Thus, keeping panels updated may prove difficult.

New multiplex panels are in development for viral, parasitic, and bacterial agents of gastrointestinal diseases, and CNS infections. A BioFire assay for usual agents of bloodstream infections was FDA approved in August 2013. At this time, it appears that the gastrointestinal panels will be direct-from-the-specimen assays, whereas the blood culture panels should be run from positive culture bottles (which may take up to 5 days to become positive). Some can detect several antibiotic resistance genes as well as infecting bacteria.

NEXT-GENERATION SEQUENCING

The advances in sequencing technology known as NextGen sequencing (NGS) have led to significant advances in basic sciences and clinical laboratory medicine, including microbiology. Currently available NGS techniques are based on using clonal amplicons for parallel multistrand sequencing. The combination of high-speed and high-throughput data analysis has made NGS an excellent tool to take clinical analysis of nucleic acid sequences to a new level. With NGS, it is possible to detect and quantify quasispecies of HIV, HCV, or HBV circulating at low levels in the blood of infected patients and to learn more about their roles in the development of resistance and associated treatment failures. This was difficult or impossible by using methods mentioned previously. Despite increasing numbers of articles on the applications of NGS, this system has not found its way into routine clinical microbiology testing because of lack of FDA approval, high cost, and availability of alternatives.[47]

NGS has significantly improved our ability to study the composition of entire communities of microorganisms (metagenomics) without organism culture. NGS simultaneously provides the sequences of genetic material from members of the entire microbial community. Analysis of these data allows determination of the relative proportions of organisms within the biome analyzed. It can also determine gene expression and metabolic pathway utilization in a microbial community. Human-microbial metagenomics studies are focused on understanding the relationship between commensal microbial communities in health and disease,[48] including cardiovascular disease.[4] NGS has also been applied to rapid investigations of outbreaks in hospital settings.[49]

MASS SPECTROSCOPY IN MICROBIOLOGY

Although "molecular diagnostics" is generally assumed to imply nucleic acid–based methods, mass spectroscopy (MS) has been used in microbiology since the 1970s. At that time, MS was used almost exclusively for the identification of anaerobes by analysis of volatile or volatilized short-chain organic acids. New MS techniques provide a general tool for the identification of microorganisms growing in colonies on culture plates. This requires 2 to 5 minutes and has the potential to improve significantly the turnaround time for microbiology culture reports and to reduce labor costs, especially when coupled with other laboratory automation that is now becoming available. Up-front costs are high, but rapidity of results can impact antibiotic usage and patient outcomes, shortening hospital stays and lowering total costs.[3]

The new technology is matrix-assisted laser desorption/ionization time of flight (MALDI TOF). Currently, there are 2 MALDI TOF instruments available in the United States for rapid identification of microorganisms. One, developed by Shimadzu Scientific Instruments (Columbia, MD) and licensed to BioMerieux (Durham, NC), has just been FDA-approved. The other can be obtained directly from its manufacturer (Bruker Daltonics, Bellerica, MA), who has also licensed it to both Siemens Healthcare Diagnostics (Tarrytown, NY) and to BD. However, the great benefit of easy, rapid, and accurate identification of microorganisms has encouraged some laboratories to purchase these systems and perform their own validations before FDA clearance.

Microorganism identification by MALDI TOF is based on the fact that each microorganism has its unique protein signature (PS). Bacterial cells are fixed to a matrix and exposed to a laser beam that releases and ionizes the proteins. These enter a vacuum column and move toward the detector based on charge and mass. The PS is checked for a match against a rapidly accumulating database derived from different genera and species of microorganisms. Different instruments have different databases.

MALDI TOF can identify microorganisms, including aerobic/anaerobic bacteria, mycobacteria, and fungi. The analysis of organisms with tougher cell walls, such as gram-positive bacteria, yeasts, and fungi, apparently requires a slight modification of procedure.[50] Hundreds of abstracts and articles attest to its ability to rapidly and accurately identify bacteria and fungi to the genus and species level.

MALDI TOF for the identification of etiologic agents of sepsis generally cannot be performed until the pathogen has first been grown in blood culture bottles and subcultured onto standard solid media. These steps are time consuming and lead to the use of broad-spectrum, empiric antibiotics. To increase speed of identification, protocols have been developed to use MALDI TOF directly from newly positive blood culture bottles.[51] Data are also accumulating illustrating the ability of MALDI TOF to identify some antibiotic-resistant organisms.[52] However, more work is needed in this area before MALDI TOF could be considered as a valid alternative to routine antibiotic susceptibility methods.

Other systems that also use MS have been tested for their ability for rapid microorganism identification. Two examples are briefly mentioned: laser-induced breakdown spectroscopy (LIBS) and Raman spectroscopy (RS). LIBS can identify microorganisms in a very short time based on determination of their elemental compositions. The system uses a strong laser beam pulse that atomizes the content of bacterial cells. Light emitted from these "high-temperature sparks" is collected and dispersed. The atoms present in the specimen are identified by peaks in the atomic emission spectrum. The ratios of the intensities of these peaks form a "spectral fingerprint" that is unique to the bacterial genus and species (LIBS spectrum). This is compared with a database to allow identification of bacterial genus/species.[53] RS can also rapidly identify bacteria to the strain level. It uses a visible or near-infrared laser that provides a reproducible molecular spectrum from the whole bacterial cell, which is unique for each bacterial species.[54]

LATE BREAKER TECHNIQUES

While this article was in preparation, 2 articles using a novel technique were published.[55,56] Chung and colleagues[55] used polystyrene beads coated with capture probe sequences common to all 16S bacterial rRNA sequences. Asymmetric PCR on the specimen was performed using 16S bacterial rRNA as a target. The PCR product was captured by the capture probes and probed with organism-specific detector probes complementary to species-specific regions of the rRNA molecules. The detector probes are covalently linked to magnetic nanoparticles. The bound magnetic nanoparticles are detected by faster relaxation of their signal in a micronuclear magnetic resonance system. The assay is carried out in a microfluidic chip, requires 2 hours and can be carried out with only 2 μL of sample. It can reportedly detect 1 bacterial cell, as well as multiple infections, and can be applied directly to blood and aspirated body fluids. It has been adapted to detect the mRNAs of *mecA* (which codes for PBP2a, the enzyme responsible for methicillin-resistance in *S aureus*), and the Panton-Valentine leukocidin, which is found in the most common of the community-associated methicillin-resistant *S aureus*. The instrumentation could be used for point of care testing.

The article by Liong and colleagues[56] focuses on the diagnosis of *M tuberculosis*. This assay is similar to the one by Chung and colleagues[55] and is also performed in a microfluidic chip. Sputum specimens are liquefied and loaded into the chip where all steps of the assay are performed, and the nuclear magnetic resonance (NMR) signal relaxation is measured at the end. The assay is also capable of detecting mutations associated with drug resistance.

If future research confirms and extends these findings, all phases of our wildest 1983 dreams may actually be coming true in 2013.

REFERENCES

1. Alexander BD, Ashley ED, Reller LB, et al. Cost savings with implementation of PNA FISH testing for identification of *Candida albicans* in blood cultures. Diagn Microbiol Infect Dis 2006;54:277–82.
2. Forrest GN, Roghmann MC, Toombs LS, et al. Peptide nucleic acid fluorescent in situ hybridization for hospital-acquired enterococcal bacteremia: delivering earlier effective antimicrobial therapy. Antimicrob Agents Chemother 2008;52: 3558–63.

3. Perez KK, Olsen RJ, Musick WL, et al. Integrating rapid pathogen identification and antimicrobial stewardship significantly decreases hospital costs. Arch Pathol Lab Med 2013;137:1247–54. Accessed September 12, 2013.

4. Karlsson FH, Fak F, Nookaew I, et al. Symptomatic atherosclerosis is associated with an altered gut metagenome. Nat Commun 2012;3:1245. http://dx.doi.org/10.1038/ncomms2266. Accessed September 12, 2013.

5. AccuProbe *Mycobacterium tuberculosis* complex culture identification test. Package Insert. Hologic Gen-Probe. Revision 2011-02. Accessed on line April 28, 2013. Available at: http://www.gen-probe.com/pdfs/pi/102896RevN.pdf.

6. García-Garrote F, Ruiz-Serrano MJ, Cosín J, et al. *Mycobacterium celatum* as a cause of disseminated infection in an AIDS patient. A case report and review of the literature. Clin Microbiol Infect 1997;3:582–4.

7. Welch DF, Guruswamy AP, Sides SJ, et al. Timely culture for mycobacteria which utilizes a microcolony method. J Clin Microbiol 1993;31:2178–84.

8. Becton Dickinson. Bacte Myco/F Sputa. Package Insert. Revision 2010/2. Accessed on line 4/20/2013. Available at: http://www.bd.com/ds/technicalCenter/inserts/PP101JAA(2011002).pdf.

9. Lie AK, Kristensen G. Human papillomavirus E6/E7 mRNA testing as a predictive marker for cervical carcinoma. Expert Rev Mol Diagn 2008;8:405–15.

10. Qiagen. Digene Hybrid Capture 2 High-Risk HPV DNA Test. Ref 5199–1220. Package insert. Accessed on line 5/2/2013. Available at: http://www.qiagen.com/resources/Download.aspx?id=(0A98CB57-25B9-48A9-9C4F-4C66D1CDA47C)&lang=en&ver=5. Accessed September 9, 2013.

11. Gravitt E, Rostich AF, Silver MI, et al. A cohort effect of the sexual revolution may be masking an increase in human papillomavirus detection at menopause in the United States. J Infect Dis 2013;207:274–80 Queried on line 4/2/2013.

12. Quiroga-Garza G, Zhou H, Mody DR. Unexpected high prevalence of HPV 90 infection in an underserved population: is it really a low-risk genotype? Arch Pathol Lab Med 2013. [Epub ahead of print]. http://dx.doi.org/10.5858/arpa.2012-0640-OA.

13. Bayer. Versant HIV-1 RNA 3.0 Assay (bDNA) Package Insert. Queried on line 4/28/2013.

14. Baumeister MA, Zhang N, Beas H, et al. A sensitive branched DNA HIV-1 signal amplification viral load technique with a single day turnaround. PLoS One 2012;7:e33295. http://dx.doi.org/10.1371/journal.pone.0033295 queried on line 4/26/2013.

15. Salimnia H, Moore EC, Crane LR, et al. Discordance between viral loads determined by Roche COBAS AMPLICOR human immunodeficiency virus type 1 monitor (version 1.5) standard and ultrasensitive assays caused by freezing patient plasma in centrifuged Becton-Dickinson vacutainer brand plasma preparation tubes. J Clin Microbiol 2005;43:4635–9.

16. Fairfax MR, Salimnia H. Beware of unusual organisms masquerading as skin contaminants. In: Azevedo L, editor. Sepsis—an ongoing and significant challenge. Rijeka (Croatia): Intech Open; 2012. p. 275–86.

17. Becton Dickinson. BD Affirm VPIII Microbial Identification Test. Package Insert. Revision of 2006/02 Queried on line 04/25/2013. Available at: http://www.bd.com/ds/technicalCenter/inserts/pkgInserts.asp#PF8.

18. Bhargava A, Mitchell R, Painter T, et al. Co-infections based upon DNA Homology: Two years experience at a Tertiary Medical Centre. Presented at ICAAC 2012. San Francisco, September 9–12, 2012.

19. Andrea SB, Chapin KC. Comparison of Aptima *Trichomonas vaginalis* transcription-mediated amplification assay and BD Affirm VPIII for detection of *T. vaginalis* in symptomatic women: performance parameters and epidemiologic implications. J Clin Microbiol 2011;49:866–9.

20. Gen-Probe. Aptima Combo 2 Assay. Package Insert. Version 2011-04. Queried on line: 05/20/2013. Available at: http://www.gen-probe.com/pdfs/pi/501799-EN-RevD.pdf.

21. Taylor SN, Van der Pol B, Lillis B, et al. Clinical evaluation of the BD ProbeTec *Chlamydia trachomatis* Qx amplified DNA assay on the BD Viper system with XTR technology. Sex Transm Dis 2011;38:603–9.

22. Cook RL, Hutchison SL, Ostergaard L, et al. Systematic review: noninvasive testing for *Chlamydia trachomatis* and *Neisseria gonorrhoeae*. Ann Intern Med 2005;142:915–25.

23. Becton Dickinson. ProbeTec *Chlamydia trachomatis* (CT) Qx Amplified DNA assay. Package insert. Version 2010/12. queried on line 5/12/2013. Available at: http://www.bd.com/ds/technicalCenter/inserts/8981498(201012).pdf.

24. Tabrizi SN, Unemo M, Limnios AE, et al. Evaluation of six commercial nucleic acid amplification tests for detection of *Neisseria gonorrhoeae* and other *Neisseria* species. J Clin Microbiol 2011;49:3610–5.

25. Cheng A, Qian Q, Kirby JE. Evaluation of the Abbott RealTime CT/NG assay in comparison to the Roche Cpbas Amplicor CT/NG Assay. J Clin Microbiol 2011; 49:1294–300.

26. Schacter J, Moncada J, Liska S, et al. Nucleic acid amplification tests in the diagnosis of chlamydial and gonococcal infections of the oropharynx and rectum in men who have sex with men. Sex Transm Dis 2008;35:637–42.

27. Moller JK, Pedersen LN, Persson K. Comparison of the Abbott RealTime CT new formulation assay with two other commercial assays for the detection of wild-type and new variant strains of *Chlamydia trachomatis*. J Clin Microbiol 2010; 48:440–3.

28. Won H, Ramachandran P, Steece R, et al. Is there evidence of the new variant *Chlamydia trachomatis* in the United States. Sex Transm Dis 2013; 40:352–3.

29. Centers for Disease Control and Prevention. Update to CDC's sexually transmitted diseases treatment guidelines, 2010: oral cephalosporins no longer a recommended treatment for gonococcal infections. MMWR Morb Mortal Wkly Rep 2012;61:590–4.

30. BD. ProbeTec Herpes Simplex Viruses (HSV 1 & 2) QxAmplified DNA Assays. Version 2012/10. Queried on line 5/20/2013. Available at: http://www.bd.com/ds/technicalCenter/inserts/8086121(01).pdf.

31. Gen-Probe. Gen-Probe Procleix Ultrio Plus Assay. 502432-REG Rev.7, as submitted to the FDA. Queried on line 5/20/2013. Available at: http://www.fda.gov/downloads/BiologicsBloodVaccines/BloodBloodProducts/ApprovedProducts/LicensedProductsBLAs/BloodDonorScreening/InfectiousDisease/UCM335285.pdf.

32. Maurin M. Real-time PCR as a diagnostic tool for bacterial diseases. Expert Rev Mol Diagn 2012;12:731–54.

33. Fairfax MR, Salimnia H. Quantitative PCR: an introduction. In: Grody WW, Strom C, Kiechle FL, et al, editors. Handbook of molecular diagnostics. London, UK: Academic Press; 2010. p. 3–14.

34. Espy MJ, Uhl P, Mitchell S, et al. Diagnosis of herpes simplex virus in the clinical laboratory by LightCycler PCR. J Clin Microbiol 2000;38:795–9.

35. Issa NC, Espy MJ, Uhl P, et al. Sequencing and resolution of amplified herpes simplex virus with intermediate melting curves as genotype 1 or 2 by light cycler PCR assay. J Clin Microbiol 2005;43:1843–5.

36. Available at: http://www.luminexcorp.com/prod/groups/public/documents/lmnxcorp/342-multicode-tech.pdf. Accessed May 12, 2013.

37. Salimnia H, Lephart PR, Asmar BI, et al. Aerosolized vaccine as an unexpected source of false positive Bordetella pertussis PCR Results. J Clin Microbiol 2012; 50:472–4.

38. Strain MC, Richmond DD. New assays for monitoring residual HIV burden in effectively treated individuals. Curr Opin HIV AIDS 2013;8:106–10.

39. Sire JM, Vray M, Merzouk M, et al. Comparative RNA quantification of HIV-1 group M and non-M with the Roche Cobas AmpliPrep/Cobas TaqMan HIV-1 v2.0 and Abbott Real-Time HIV-1 PCR assays. J Acquir Immune Defic Syndr 2011;56(3):239–43.

40. Wojewoda CM, Shalinger T, Harmon ML, et al. Comparison of Roche Cobas AmpliPrep/Cobas TaqMan HIV-1 test version 2.0 (CAP/CTM v2.0) with other real-time PCR assays in HIV monitoring and follow-up of low-level viral loads. J Virol Methods 2013;187:1–5.

41. Babady NE, Mead P, Stiles J, et al. Comparison of the Luminex xTAG RVP Fast-Assay with the Idaho Technology FilmArray RP Assay for detection of respiratory viruses in pediatric patients at a cancer hospital. J Clin Microbiol 2012;50: 2282–8.

42. McGrath EJ, Thomas R, Asmar B, et al. Detection of respiratory co-infections in pediatric patients using a small volume polymerase chain reaction array respiratory panel: more evidence for combined droplet and contact isolation. Am J Infect Control 2013;41:868–73. Queried on line 4/1/2013.

43. Popowich EB, O'Niel SS, Miller MM. Comparison of the Biofire FilmArray RP, Genmark eSensor RBP, Luminex xTAG RVPv1, and Luminex xTAG RVP Fast multiplex assays for detection of respiratory viruses. J Clin Microbiol 2013;51(5):1528–33. http://dx.doi.org/10.1128/JCM.03368-12. Accessed 5/16/2012.

44. Mahoney JB. Nucleic acid amplification-based diagnosis of respiratory virus infections. Expert Rev Anti Infect Ther 2010;8(11):1273–92. Available at: http://dx.doi.org/10.1586/eri.10.121. Accessed May 16, 2013.

45. de Groot RJ, Baker SC, Baric RS, et al. Middle East Respiratory Syndrome Coronavirus (MERS-CoV); announcement of the coronavirus study group. J Virol 2013;87:7790–2. http://dx.doi.org/10.1128/JVI.0244-13 queried on 5/20/2013.

46. Liu F, Shi W, Shi Y, et al. Origin and diversity of novel influenza A7N9 viruses causing human infection; phylogenetic, structural and coalescent analyses. Lancet 2013;381:1926–32. Accessed 5/21/13.

47. Capobianchi MR, Giombini E, Rozera G. Next-generation sequencing technology in clinical virology. Clin Microbiol Infect 2013;19(1):15–22. http://dx.doi.org/10.1111/1469-0691.12056.

48. Song S, Jarvie T, Hattori M. Our second genome-human metagenome: how next-generation sequencer changes our life through microbiology. Adv Microb Physiol 2013;62:119–44. http://dx.doi.org/10.1016/B978-0-12-410515-7.00003-2.

49. Sherry NL, Porter JL, Seemann T, et al. Outbreak investigation using high-throughput genome sequencing within a diagnostic microbiology laboratory. J Clin Microbiol 2013;51:1396–401. http://dx.doi.org/10.1128/JCM.03332-12.

50. Theel ES, Schmitt BH, Hall L, et al. Formic acid-based direct, on-plate testing of yeast and corynebacterium species by Bruker Biotyper matrix-assisted laser

desorption ionization-time of flight mass spectrometry. J Clin Microbiol 2012;50: 3093–5. http://dx.doi.org/10.1128/JCM.01045-12.

51. March-Rosselló GA, Muñoz-Moreno MF, García-Loygorri-Jordán de Urriés MC, et al. A differential centrifugation protocol and validation criterion for enhancing mass spectrometry (MALDI-TOF) results in microbial identification using blood culture growth bottles. Eur J Clin Microbiol Infect Dis 2013;32:699–704. http:// dx.doi.org/10.1007/s10096-012-1797-1.

52. Wimmer JL, Long SW, Cernoch P, et al. Strategy for rapid identification and anti-biotic susceptibility testing of gram-negative bacteria directly recovered from positive blood cultures using the Bruker MALDI Biotyper and the BD Phoenix system. J Clin Microbiol 2012;50(7):2452–4.

53. Rehse SJ, Salimnia H, Miziolek AW, et al. Laser-induced breakdown spectros-copy (LIBS): an overview of recent progress and future potential for biomedical applications. J Med Eng Technol 2012;36:77–89.

54. Hamasha K, Mohaidat QI, Putnam RA, et al. Sensitive and specific discrimina-tion of pathogenic and nonpathogenic *Escherichia coli* using Raman spectros-copy—a comparison of two multivariate analysis techniques. Biomed Opt Express 2013;4:481–9.

55. Chung HJ, Castro CM, Im H, et al. A magneto-DNA nanoparticle system for rapid detection and phenotyping of bacteria. Nat Nanotechnol 2013;8:369–75. http://dx.doi.org/10.1038/nnano.2013.70. Accessed 5/20/2013.

56. Liong M, Hoang AN, Chung J, et al. Magnetic barcode assay for genetic detec-tion of pathogens. Nat Commun 2013;4. http://dx.doi.org/10.1038/ncomms2745. Accessed 5/19/2013.

Molecular Pathology in Transfusion Medicine

Matthew B. Elkins, MD, PhD[a,*], Robertson D. Davenport, MD[b],
Barbara A. O'Malley, MD[c], Martin H. Bluth, MD, PhD[d]

KEYWORDS

- Genotype • Phenotype • Serology • Antigen • Antibody • Blood donors
- Transfusion • Red blood cells • Platelets

KEY POINTS

- Virtually all the red cell and platelet antigen systems have been characterized at the molecular level.
- Highly reliable methods for red cell and platelet antigen genotyping are now available.
- Genotyping is a useful adjunct to traditional serology and can help resolve complex serologic problems.
- Although red cell and platelet phenotype can be inferred from genotype, knowledge of the molecular bases is essential for accurate assignment.
- Genotyping of blood donors is an effective method of identifying antigen negative and/or particularly rare donors.
- Cell-free DNA analysis provides a promising noninvasive method of assessing fetal genotypes of blood group alloantigens.

OVERVIEW

Testing performed in transfusion medicine focuses on detection of antigens expressed on the cell membrane of red blood cells (RBC) and/or platelets and the detection of antibodies against RBC or platelet antigens in a patient's plasma. Detection of these antigens and antibodies are critical because RBC or platelet units that are positive for a given antigen and that are transfused into a patient who has antibodies against that specific antigen may cause decreased blood product survival, hemolytic transfusion reactions, hyperhemolysis reactions, and even death.

[a] Department of Pathology, Upstate Medical University, 750 East Adams Street, Syracuse, NY 13210, USA; [b] Department of Pathology, University of Michigan Health System, UH 2G332, 1500 East Medical Center Drive, Ann Arbor, MI 48109-5054, USA; [c] Department of Pathology, Detroit Medical Center, Wayne State University, 3990 John R. Street, Detroit, MI 48201, USA; [d] Karmanos Cancer Institute, Detroit Medical Center, Wayne State University School of Medicine, 3990 John R. Street, Detroit, MI 48201, USA
* Corresponding author.
E-mail address: ElkinsM@upstate.edu

Clin Lab Med 33 (2013) 805–816
http://dx.doi.org/10.1016/j.cll.2013.08.004
0272-2712/13/$ – see front matter © 2013 Elsevier Inc. All rights reserved.

RBC and platelet antigens and antibodies are traditionally detected using serologic assays. These assays overwhelmingly use hemagglutination to indicate the presence of an antibody in the tested serum and the presence of the antigen on the tested RBC or platelet product. For example, forward typing of a patient's RBC antigens is performed by combining the patient's RBCs with known anti-A, anti-B, and anti-D antisera. Any reaction resulting in agglutinated RBCs suggests that the RBCs have that antigen on their surface (eg, agglutination in anti-A reaction suggests the presence of the A antigen on the RBC membrane). To cause agglutination, the assays rely on the agglutination capability of the tested antibodies (eg, ABO testing) for the IgM class and secondary antibodies (eg, anti-human globulin antibodies, anti-C3 antibodies) for the IgG class.

ADVANTAGES OF MOLECULAR TESTING

Molecular testing is complementary to traditional serologic testing used for most transfusion medicine testing.[1] Molecular testing does not replace serologic testing, and serologic testing is still very much the backbone of transfusion medicine testing. Serologic testing is well characterized, sensitive enough to find and identify most clinically significant alloantibodies, and useful for most patient situations. However, serologic testing is limited in specific patients and situations. These include:

Patients with confounding antibodies (warm or cold autoantibodies, cold agglutinins, neonate with passive maternal antibodies)

Patients with antigens or antibodies for which testing antibodies or antisera are not available (partial or variant antigens, rare antigens, high-incidence antigens)

Patients with a mixture of circulating RBCs or plasma (recently transfused, after bone marrow transplant, after plasmapheresis)

Patients in whom antigen zygosity needs to be determined

Mass screenings of blood donors.

In each of these situations, serologic testing may be of limited sensitivity and specificity or may be prohibitive in time, effort, or cost.

Obscuring autoantibodies or multiple alloantibodies can cause unexpected agglutination in test reactions. This can result in an inability to rule out alloantibody possibilities, making it difficult or impossible to identify any clinically significant alloantibodies in the patient's serum. Antibodies against low-incidence antigens may not be effectively identified because of the limited availability of antisera and antigen-positive test RBCs. Similarly, antibodies to high-incidence antigens may be difficult to identify because of the lack of commercially available antisera or antigen-negative reagent red cells. In patients who have received multiple RBC transfusions, the transfused RBCs may obscure the presence or absence of antigens of interest on the patient's native RBCs. Likewise, the serum of patients receiving multiple plasma transfusions or automated plasma exchange cannot be evaluated for antibodies from the patient's native immune system because of obscuring or dilution by the transfused plasma. For many RBC or platelet antigens, the phenotypes of homozygous and heterozygous patients are often indistinguishable by serologic means. For example, although there is the concept of "dosing," observing differences in the strength of hemagglutination when reagent RBCs have homozygous versus heterozygous expression of a given phenotype, RBCs that only have one copy of a specific allele can look the same as RBCs with two copies. Mass screenings of the antigen status of RBCs or platelets is a daunting task using serologic methods because of the poor scalability, considerable cost, and limited automation options.

Thus, each blood component unit must be individually tested for each antigen using relatively labor-intensive techniques.

For each of these situations, molecular testing may allow determination of antigens expressed by the patient or donor. Determination of the antigens expressed by a patient also may be used presumptively to predict which alloantibodies can be produced by the patient (because an individual can make alloantibodies only against antigens that the individual lacks).

LIMITATIONS OF MOLECULAR TESTING

There are limitations to the application of molecular testing in transfusion medicine. Primarily, molecular testing provides information on the genotype of the patient and, as such, cannot determine the specificities of any antibodies within a patient's serum. Molecular testing can only determine the antigens that the patient makes and, therefore, which antigen specificities that patient could theoretically make antibodies against. A patient with unknown antibody (or antibodies) may be molecularly typed to express D, C, e, and Jk(a), but not express c, E, and Jk(b). Based solely on this information, antibodies in the patient's serum could be specific to any one or multiples of the antigens c, E, Jk(b), or to another RBC antigen not tested by the molecular assay. Serologic testing is required to determine the specificity (or specificities) of the patient's antibody (or antibodies).

Molecular testing is promulgated on the frequency of anticipated polymorphism common within a population. As such, it is limited in detection of genes with an abundance of alleles (eg, ABO system) and antigens for which the coding gene is not known. Further, molecular testing assays performed using allele-specific polymerase chain reaction (PCR) in which amplicon identification is made based on size, will not detect point mutations, inversions, or other alterations of the DNA sequence that do not alter either the targeted primer sites or the amplicon size. At this point, most institutions are batching molecular testing, thus increasing turn-around time, with the result that, at this point, molecular testing may be significantly slower than serologic testing for uncomplicated patients. Finally, if possible, molecular testing results should be confirmed using serologic testing because genetic determinants outside the gene tested (eg, promoters) may affect the expression of that antigen. This results in a patient or donor being labeled as "positive" for an antigen when he or she does not actually express that antigen.[2] An example is the D—haplotype in which there is no apparent expression by serologic testing of any of the RHCE antigens in a D-positive person despite the presence of the RHCE genes. This phenotype is due to a single nucleotide (907C) deletion in exon 6 that introduces a premature stop codon, which results in the silencing of the RHCE genes.[3] Similarly, alleles that vary expression depending on their cis or trans orientation may also lead to discrepant results between phenotype and genotype testing approaches.

MOLECULAR TECHNIQUES USED IN TRANSFUSION MEDICINE

The molecular techniques currently used for testing in transfusion medicine are all based on amplification of sequences from the DNA of the patient or donor. The targets of testing are the genes that determine the production of red blood cell or platelet antigenic determinants. These techniques are used as an adjunct to serologic testing in determining either the antigens expressed on the cell membranes of donated blood products or antigens not expressed on the cell membranes of blood transfusion recipients. These techniques help determine which antigens the recipient may make antibodies against, thereby forecasting possible incompatibilities for future transfusions.

Transfusion testing is particularly amenable to molecular methods because most assays evaluate constitutional genetic expression (germline expression), thus avoiding the sensitivity problems seen in some molecular testing targeted toward somatic mutations within a background of germline genes.

Current testing methodologies include various permutations of PCR, restriction fragment length polymorphism (RFLP), Sanger sequencing, and high-throughput multiplex PCR. The most commonly used testing methods are PCR with allele-specific primers and detection of amplicons by traditional gel or capillary electrophoresis, using either commercially available kits, or published or in-house protocols.[4,5] The downside of this approach is that a separate PCR reaction must be set up and a separate detection assay (gel or capillary electrophoresis) must be run for each antigen to be evaluated. This results in a relatively slow, labor-intensive process. However, in a practice with a low volume of molecular testing, these assays require relatively low investment in supporting technology.

One of the approaches to minimize the labor required and increase the information output from a single assay is to multiplex the molecular assays, using multiple PCR primer sets in a single reaction to assay for multiple allele-specific RBC antigen genes. There are various multiplex approaches, each of which uses a specific detection method to report which allelic amplicons are produced by the multiplex PCR. Three commercially available systems using multiplexed PCR are the HEA BeadChip system and LifeCodes RBC (both Immucor Inc, Norcross, GA, USA), and the BLOODchip (Progenika Inc, Medford, MA, USA).[6–8] In the BeadChip system, the resultant PCR amplicons are hybridized to allele-specific probes bound to fluorescent beads. If the sequences are a match, the probe will be extended by PCR and the resultant increase in fluorescence is detected. The pattern of fluorescence of these beads is then interpreted to determine which PCR products are present and, therefore, which genes are present in the patient's DNA. In the BLOODchip system, the amplicons are fragmented and specifically labeled with fluorophores. The labeled fragments are then hybridized to allele-specific DNA probes bound to an array and the resultant fluorescence pattern is interrogated to determine the presence of amplicons for each antigen. The LifeCodes system uses multiplexed RBC antigen allele-specific polymorphisms, which are detected using a fluorescent capture bead platform.[9] Using this system, a single multiplexed PCR reaction may be used to determine the genotype for Rh, Kell, Kidd, Duffy, MNS, and Dombrock antigen groups. A second PCR multiplex may be used to determine the genotype for Colton, Dombrock, Scianna, Lutheran, Diego, Landsteiner-Wiener (LW), Cartwright, Knops, and Cromer antigen groups. Following PCR, the amplicon products are incubated with fluorescent beads to which oligonucleotide probes are bound. The probes selectively bind the PCR products for each antigen allele. The DNA-bound beads are then detected using a flow cytometer. Using the multiplexed PCR reactions and a single flow cytometer run to detect approximately 25 antigen single nucleotide polymorphisms (SNPs) greatly increases the efficiency of molecular assays compared with a PCR reaction with a detection assay for each antigen SNP product.

Most RBC antigens have a limited array of alleles, which make them amenable to allele-specific PCR. However, some genes have a larger genetic variation (eg, Rh genes) and DNA sequencing may be used to determine the specific genetic variation present. Typically, Sanger sequencing is used, although next-generation sequencing is being explored for application to transfusion medicine testing. Sanger sequencing is performed using tagged terminating nucleotides in a single-direction PCR. The PCR products are then evaluated using electrophoresis, either gel or capillary, with the length of each product correlating with the position of the terminating base.

TERMINOLOGY AND NOTATION

The results of molecular testing for transfusion medicine may be reported at diverse levels of detail using various notation strategies. Additionally, molecular testing results may be reported either as the expressed phenotype or as the genotype, although current notation does not differentiate phenotype from genotype. For example, molecular testing may be done for the C698T point mutation resulting in the T193M amino acid substitution on the Kell gene, which results in the antigen commonly referred to simply as "K" or "Kell."[10] If this testing yields a positive result, the result may be reported as "positive for K," "positive for Kell," "heterozygous for Kell," "positive for C698T," "positive for T193M," and so forth. There are no current, widely accepted standards about how this result should be reported. One recent attempt at this standardization has been made by the International Society of Blood Transfusion, most recently referenced by Storry and colleagues[11] in 2011. The Society's complete guidelines may be found at http://www.isbtweb.org/working-parties/red-cell-immunogenetics-and-blood-group-terminology/blood-group-terminology/. These guidelines provide suggestions for naming conventions of genotype, phenotype, and antigen status for current RBC antigens, as well as guidelines for newly identified antigens.

RED CELL ANTIGEN EXPRESSION

The molecular basis of virtually all the known blood group antigens has now been established. Blood group polymorphisms arise from a variety of genetic mechanisms, including SNPs, single nucleotide deletion, gene deletion, sequence duplication, and intergenic recombination. Most antigens are the result of SNPs. The most commonly tested, clinically significant SNPs are listed in **Table 1**. Deletion of the RHD gene is the most common basis for the Rh-negative phenotype. Homozygous deletion of GYPB also accounts for the S-s-U- phenotype. Deletion of a single nucleotide results in a frame shift that may introduce a stop codon, and is responsible for the common O alleles and for the A2 allele of the ABO system. Sequence duplication with introduction of a nonsense mutation is responsible for the inactive RHD gene (RHDΨ) common among Rh-negative African Americans.

Knowledge of red cell phenotype is essential for provision of compatible blood with the recipient who has produced clinically significant antibodies, and is an important part of red cell antibody identification. Red cell phenotype is determined by immunohematologic methods. However, these methods are limited by availability of reliable antisera, are inherently subjective, and are difficult to perform when the patient was recently transfused or has a positive direct antiglobulin test. In most cases, red cell phenotype can be inferred from genotype and is a valuable adjunct to, or possible substitute for, phenotyping. The most commonly tested blood group genotypes are listed in **Table 1**. Genotyping is highly reliable and can be automated. However, phenotyping may still be preferable for some antigens, for instance those with numerous allelic variations such as ABO and Rh(D), which can be rapidly determined in most patients using inexpensive, readily available immunohematology methods.

The A and B determinants are carbohydrate structures, present on some red cell membrane glycoproteins and glycolipids, which result from the action of glycosyltransferases. The most common ABO alleles differ at 6 positions with exons 6 and 7, resulting in the A-transferase (N-acetylgalactosaminyltransferase), B-transferase (galactosyltransferase), or a nonfunctional product. However, more than 180 ABO alleles have been described to date.[12] In addition, the acceptor substrate for the A- and B-transferases is the H antigen, which is produced by transferases

Table 1			
Genetic basis of common blood group antigens			
Blood Group System	**HUGO Gene Name**	**Antigens**	**Nucleotide Changes**
MNS	GYPA	M/N	60C>T
			72G>A
	GYPB	S/s	243T>C
Rh	RHCE	C/c	178A>C
			203G>A
			307T>C
		E/e	676C>G
Lutheran	BCAM	Lu(a/b)	230G>A
Kell	KEL	K/k	698T>C
		Kp(a/b)	961T>C
		Js(a/b)	1910C>T
Duffy	DARC	Fy(a/b)	125G>A
		Fy(a-b-)	−33T>C
Kidd	SLC14A1	Jk(a/b)	838G>A
Diego	SLC4A1	Di(a/b)	2561T>C
		Wr(a/b)	1972A>G
Cartwright	ACHE	Yt(a/b)	1057C>A
Dombrock	DO	Do(a/b)	378C>T
			624T>C
			79A>G
		Hy(±)	323G>T
		Jo(a+/a−)	350C>T
Colton	AQP1	Co(a/b)	134C>T
LW	ICAM4	LW(a/b)	308A>G
Cromer	CD55	Cr(a+/a−)	679G>C
Knopps	CR1	Kn(a/b)	4681G>A
		McC(a/b)	4768A>G
		Sl(a)	4828T>A

Data from Reid ME, Lomas-Francis C. The blood group antigens fact book. 2nd edition. Elsevier; 2004; and Blood group antigen gene mutation database. Available at: http://www.ncbi.nlm.nih.gov/projects/gv/mhc/xslcgi.cgi?cmd=bgmut/home. Accessed April 16, 2013.

encoded by the tissue-specific genes FUT1 and FUT2. Although the H-negative phenotype is rare, it is responsible for a group O phenotype (Oh or Bombay) regardless of the alleles at the ABO locus. For these reasons, the value of ABO genotyping is largely for resolution of unusual ABO types.

Rh is genetically the most complex blood group system. The antigens of the Rh system are encoded by two closely linked genes, RHD and RHCE. RHD encodes the many epitopes of the D antigen. The most common genetic bases of the Rh-negative phenotype are deletion of RHD and the presence of a frameshift mutation resulting in a premature stop codon. Genotyping for RHD is largely reserved for resolution of some weak or partial D phenotypes.

Beyond the ABO and D antigens, most of the common clinically significant red cell antigens result from SNPs (see **Table 1**). The MNS antigens are present on glycophorins A and B (GPA and GPB), which are products of two closely linked homologous genes GYPA and GYPB of the glycophorin gene family, each present in two different allelic forms.[13] GPA and GPB show a high degree of sequence homology. GPA carries the epitopes for the MN blood groups, and GPB carries the epitopes for the Ss blood groups. Gene rearrangements are a prevailing mechanism for the observed DNA variation resulting in variant GPA and GPB alleles.[14] Numerous variant alleles exist that are common in some populations and may be clinically significant.

The Kell system consists of 25 antigens, which include six pairs of antithetical antigens. Each Kell antigen is determined by single nucleotide point mutations of the KEL gene encoding the Kell glycoprotein. There is considerable variation in the incidence of Kell antigens between ethnic populations.[15] On the red cell membrane, the Kell glycoprotein is covalently linked to the XK protein, which carries the Kx blood group. Weak expression of Kell antigens can be inherited or acquired and transient. Inherited weak expression occurs in the McLeod phenotype (absence of XK protein), the Leach phenotype (lack of a portion of glycophorin C), and some Gerbich-negative phenotypes (lack of all or portions of glycophorins C or D).

The Duffy blood group system comprises two common antithetical antigens and two high-incidence antigens.[15] The Duffy glycoprotein is functionally significant for its ability to bind multiple chemokines, known as Duffy antigen chemokine receptor (DARC). It is also the receptor exploited by Plasmodium vivax merozoites for entry into red cells. Because of selective pressure due to malaria, the Duffy null phenotype is common in some populations. The molecular basis of the Fy(a–b–) phenotype found in African Americans is an SNP in the promoter region (−33 T>C), which disrupts a binding site for the erythroid transcription factor GATA-1 with resultant loss of DARC expression on red cells. Because the erythroid promoter controls expression only in erythroid cells, DARC expression on endothelium is normal. To date, all alleles carrying the mutated GATA box have been shown to carry FYB, therefore Fy(b) is expressed on their nonerythroid tissues. This explains why Fy(a–b–) individuals can make anti-Fy(a) but not anti-Fy(b).

The Kidd blood group system is relatively simple with two antithetical antigens resulting from an SNP. In addition, a high-incidence antigen, Jk3, is absent in the null phenotype. The Kidd null phenotype results from two different genetic backgrounds: homozygous inheritance of a silent allele or inheritance of a dominant inhibitor gene In(Jk) unlinked to the Kidd locus SLC14A.[16]

The Diego system antigenic determinants are carried on the anion exchange multipass membrane glycoprotein Band 3. The Diego blood group system comprises 21 antigens, of which two antithetical pairs, Di(a/b) and Wr(a/b), are commonly significant.[17] Di(b) and Wr(b) are high-incidence antigens, whereas the other Diego systems antigens are low-incidence. The Yt blood group system (sometimes incorrectly referred to as the Cartwright system) consists of two antithetical antigens encoded by an SNP that are carried on acetylcholinesterase glycoprotein (ACHE). The Yt(b) antigen has moderately low incidence the United States, but is common in the Israeli population. Because ACHE is GPI-linked to the red cell membrane, red cells of patients with paroxysmal nocturnal hemoglobinemia lack Yt antigens, as well as Cromer antigens.[18]

The Dombrock blood group system comprises an antithetical pair, Do(a/b), and the high-incidence antigens Hy and Jo to which antithetical antigens have not been identified. Although anti-Do(a) and anti-Do(b) are uncommon, they may cause hemolytic transfusion reactions. Genotyping is essential to identify compatible blood donors because reliable reagent Dombrock antisera are extremely rare.

The Colton blood group system comprises an antithetical pair, Co(a/b), and a high-incidence antigen Co3, carried on the aquaporin water channel protein AQP1. Absence of Co3 results in the null phenotype, Co(a–b–), which has only been described in rare individuals.

The LW blood group system comprises an antithetical pair, LW(a/b), carried on the intracellular adhesion molecule ICAM-4. Expression of LW antigens is strongly influenced by the presence or absence of Rh proteins, so that anti-Lw(a) may be confused with anti-D. Genotyping can be very helpful in making this distinction correctly.

The Cromer blood group system comprises 12 high-incidence and 3 low-incidence antigens that are carried on CD55, the complement regulatory protein decay accelerating factor.[19] The Cr(a-) phenotype is found mainly in the African American population, although it is still rare. The antithetical antigens to Cr(a) has not been identified. The rare Cromer null phenotype, also termed Inab, is associated with lack of CD55 on red cells. In contrast to patients with paroxysmal nocturnal hemoglobinuria, Inab red cells are resistant to complement-mediated lysis. The molecular basis of the Inab phenotype is an SNP or introduction of an alternate splice site, which results in a premature stop codon.

The Knops blood group system contains eight antigens that are carried on complement receptor 1 (CR1).[20] In the white population, McC(b) and Sl(a) are low-incidence but in the African American population they are common. Antibodies to Knops antigens are clinically insignificant, but are often encountered in pretransfusion testing as so-called high-titer, low-avidity antibodies (HTLA). HTLA often demonstrate observable hemagglutination through serial dilutions and can complicate the immunohematology workup when there is suspicion of an underlying clinically significant antibody. In such cases, genotyping can be a very useful adjunct in identification and in excluding clinically significant specificities.

PLATELET ANTIGEN EXPRESSION

Platelets carry antigens of importance to the transfusion medicine, including ABO, human leukocyte antigens (HLA) class I, and platelet-specific antigens. The antigens whose expression are restricted to platelets, and as such must be investigated separately from the RBC antigens, are grouped into the human platelet antigens (HPA) nomenclature system (**Table 2**).[21] To date, 33 HPA have been defined at the molecular level. Six biallelic HPA pairs (HPA-1a/1b, -2a/2b, -3a/3b, -4a/4b, -5a/5b, -15a/15b) have been identified, with the higher frequency allele being designated with a lowercase "a," Antigens for which the corresponding allele has not been defined serologically are designated by "w" (workshop).

Identification of platelet antigens by phenotype is more difficult than red cell phenotyping. The most commonly used method is flow cytometry. However, this requires specialized instrumentation. In addition, high-quality antisera are difficult to obtain. Most human sera containing platelet antibodies also contain HLA class I antibodies, or are multispecific. Antisera for low-frequency antigens are very rare. For these reasons, genotyping has largely replaced phenotyping as a means of HPA determination.

A variety of molecular methods can be used for HPA genotyping. Because almost all of HPA arise from single base substitutions, the most commonly used method for HPA genotyping is PCR DNA amplification using oligonucleotide sequence-specific primers (PCR-SSP). The amplification conditions must be optimized for each specific primer set. PCR-SSP is commonly used because it is a relatively simple and inexpensive procedure; however, post-PCR processing steps are required. Melting curve analysis is another commonly used method for HPA genotyping. In this technique, PCR amplification of DNA containing the platelet SNP of interest is performed using flanking primers. The product is detected using two differently labeled fluorescent oligonucleotide probes that bind to adjacent sequences on the patient's DNA near the SNP. Binding of both probes is detected by fluorescence energy transfer (FRET). The instrument takes a series of readings at increasing temperatures that

Table 2
Genetic basis of human platelet antigens

Antigen	Glycoprotein	HGNC Identifier	Chromosome	Nucleotide Change	Mature Protein
HPA-1a/1b	GPIIIa	ITGB3	17	176T>C	L33P
HPA-2a/2b	GPIba	GP1BA	17	482C>T	T145M
HPA-3a/3b	GPIIb	ITGA2B	17	2621T>G	I843S
HPA-4a/4b	GPIIIa	ITGB3	17	506G>A	R143Q
HPA-5a/5b	GPIa	ITGA2	5	1600G>A	E505K
HPA-6w	GPIIIa	ITGB3	17	1544G>A	R489Q
HPA-7w	GPIIIa	ITGB3	17	1297C>G	P407A
HPA-8w	GPIIIa	ITGB3	17	1984C>T	R636C
HPA-9w	GPIIb	ITGA2B	17	2602G>A	V837M
HPA-10w	GPIIIa	ITGB3	17	263G>A	R62Q
HPA-11w	GPIIIa	ITGB3	17	1976G>A	R633H
HPA-12w	GPIbb	GP1BB	22	119G>A	G15E
HPA-13w	GPIa	ITGA2	5	2483C>T	T799M
HPA-14w	GPIIIa	ITGB3	17	1909_1911delAAG	K611del
HPA-15a/15b	CD109	CD109	6	2108C>A	S682Y
HPA-16w	GPIIIa	ITGB3	17	497C>T	T140I
HPA-17w	GPIIIa	ITGB3	17	662C>T	T195M
HPA-18w	GP1a	ITGA2	5	2235G>T	Q716H
HPA-19w	GPIIIa	ITGB3	17	487A>C	K137Q
HPA-20w	GPIIb	ITGA2B	17	1949C>T	T619M
HPA-21w	GPIIIa	ITGB3	17	1960G>A	E628K
HPA-22bw	GPIIb	ITGA2B	17	584A>C	K164T
HPA-23bw	GPIIIa	ITGB3	17	1942C>T	R622W
HPA-24bw	GPIIb	ITGA2B	17	1508G>A	S472N
HPA-25bw	GPIa	ITGA2	5	3347C>T	T1087M
HPA-26bw	GPIIIa	ITGB3	17	1818G>T	K580N
HPA-27bw	GPIIb	ITGA2B	17	2614C>A	L841M

Abbreviation: HGNC, Human Genome Organization Gene Nomenclature Committee.
Data from European Molecular Biology Institute–European Bioinformatics Institute. IPD-HPA database. Available at: http://www.ebi.ac.uk/ipd/hpa/. Accessed April 16, 2013.

allow the probes to dissociate, or "melt off" at different temperatures, generating a melting curve, the shape of which depends on the presence or absence of the SNP of interest. A third method is the 50-nuclease assay, or TaqMan, real-time PCR assay (RT-PCR). This uses two sequence-specific, single-stranded DNA probes (TaqMan probes) 5′ labeled with different reporter fluorophores, and a quencher molecule attached to the 3′ ends. The probes are designed to bind to the platelet SNP of interest on the DNA template. When bound in close proximity to the quencher, the fluorescence of the reporter is reduced through FRET. Practical genotyping for large-scale screening, such as blood donor or NAIT screening, requires high-throughput methods. Several multiplex, PCR-based, high-throughput systems using glass slide microarrays, microplate arrays, and liquid bead arrays have been described.[22–25]

The most common clinical situations in which platelet antigen determination are used are fetal and neonatal alloimmune thrombocytopenia (FNAIT) and posttransfusion purpura (PTP). Less common uses include evaluation of platelet transfusion refractoriness, immune thrombocytopenia (ITP), and drug-induced immune thrombocytopenia. In FNAIT, maternal IgG alloantibodies to platelet antigens cross the placenta causing fetal, and subsequently neonatal, thrombocytopenia. Determination that the mother is negative for the implicated platelet antigen establishes that the pregnancy is at risk; however, it does not necessarily indicate that the pregnancy is affected. Determination that the father is homozygous for the implicated antigen, or that the fetus is positive, identifies the pregnancy as high-risk. PTP is a rare complication of transfusion in which alloimmunization to a platelet antigen is coincident with a period of severe thrombocytopenia. Determination that the patient is negative for the implicated platelet antigen establishes the diagnosis. For both of these applications, genotyping has distinct advantages compared with phenotyping, because it does not require platelets and may be performed on somatic DNA obtained from peripheral blood, buccal swab, or amniotic fluid. Platelet antigen determination has a limited role in management of the multitransfused platelet refractory patient because antibodies to HPA are rare in this setting and, when they do occur, are usually in conjunction with HLA antibodies.[26] In ITP and drug-induced immune thrombocytopenia, antibody identification rarely requires HPA typing.

CELL FREE NUCLEIC ACID TESTING

During the past decade, the discovery of cell-free nucleic acids in serum, plasma, urine, or other body fluids has promoted investigation of genes encoding proteins as a means to detect diseases with potentially greater sensitivity. Normally, DNA is isolated from tissue through standard procedures using phenol chloroform extraction followed by ethanol precipitation. However, DNA can also be obtained directly from serum, plasma, or other body fluids by centrifugation, separating it from cells and platelets and subsequently interrogated using amplification methods such as RT-PCR or other detection methods.[27] The use of cell-free nucleic acid interrogation also has application to the discipline of transfusion medicine.[28] Studies on fetal *RHD* typing in maternal plasma samples of pregnant women in different periods of pregnancy have been reported.[29–31] Studies by Brojer and colleagues[29] found that maternal plasma may be confidently used as a sample source for detection of fetal RHD genotyping (99.6% predictive value) after one set of RT-PCR procedures, with the understanding that implementation of additional polymorphisms can increase the predictive value to 100%. Recent studies on noninvasive genotyping of other blood group alloantigens (D, c, E, and Kell) have also been reported.[32] In the setting of FNAIT, genotyping for fetal platelet antigens can also be performed on cell-free fetal DNA extracted from maternal plasma.[33,34]

REFERENCES

1. Reid ME. Transfusion in the age of molecular diagnostics. Hematology Am Soc Hematol Educ Program 2009;171–7.
2. Singleton BK, Frayne J, Anstee DJ. Blood group phenotypes resulting from mutations in erythroid transcription factors. Curr Opin Hematol 2012;19:486–93.
3. Westhoff CM, Vege S, Nickle P, et al. Nucleotide deletion in RHCE*cE (907delC) is responsible for a D- - haplotype in Hispanics. Transfusion 2011;51:2142–7.
4. Daniels G, van der Schoot CE, Olsson ML. Report of the fourth International Workshop on molecular blood group genotyping. Vox Sang 2011;101:327–32.

5. Monteiro F, Tavares G, Ferreira M, et al. Technologies involved in molecular blood group genotyping. ISBT Sci Ser 2011;6:1–6.
6. Immucor, Inc. Molecular immunohematology. Available at: http://www.immucor.com/Global/Products/Pages/Molecular.aspx. Accessed April 16, 2013.
7. Progenika, Inc. BLOODchip reference. Available at: http://www.progenika.com/eu/index.php?option=com_content&task=view&id=302&Itemid=384. Accessed April 16, 2013.
8. Immucor, Inc. LIFECODES. Available at: http://www.immucor.com/en-us/Pages/LIFECODES.aspx. Accessed April 16, 2013.
9. Drago F, Karpasitou K, Poli F. Microarray beads for identifying blood group single nucleotide polymorphisms. Transfus Med Hemother 2009;36:157–60.
10. Lee S. Molecular basis of Kell blood group phenotypes. Vox Sang 1997;73: 1–11.
11. Storry JR, Castilho L, Daniels G, et al. International Society of Blood Transfusion Working Party on red cell immunogenetics and blood group terminology: Berlin report. Vox Sang 2011;101:77–82.
12. ABO Blood Group System. Available at: http://www.ncbi.nlm.nih.gov/projects/gv/mhc/xslcgi.cgi?cmd=bgmut/systems_info&system=abo. Accessed April 16, 2013.
13. Reid ME. MNS blood group system: a review. Immunohematology 2009;25: 95–101.
14. Shih MC, Yang LH, Wang NM, et al. Genomic typing of human red cell miltenberger glycophorins in a Taiwanese population. Transfusion 2000;40:54–61.
15. Westhoff CM, Reid ME. Review: the Kell, Duffy, and Kidd blood group systems. Immunohematology 2004;20:37–49.
16. Fröhlich O, Macey RI, Edwards-Moulds J, et al. Urea transport deficiency in Jk(a–b–) erythrocytes. Am J Physiol 1991;260:C778–83.
17. Byrne KM, Byrne PC. Review: other blood group systems—Diego, Yt, Xg, Scianna, Dombrock, Colton, Landsteiner-Wiener, and Indian. Immunohematology 2004;20:50–8.
18. Telen MJ. Glycosyl phosphatidylinositol-linked blood group antigens and paroxysmal nocturnal hemoglobinuria. Transfus Clin Biol 1995;2:277–90.
19. Storry JR, Reid ME, Yazer MH. The Cromer blood group system: a review. Immunohematology 2010;26(3):109–18.
20. Moulds JM. The Knops blood-group system: a review. Immunohematology 2010; 26(1):2–7.
21. European Molecular Biology Institute–European Bioinformatics Institute. IPD-HPA database. Available at: http://www.ebi.ac.uk/ipd/hpa/. Accessed April 16, 2013.
22. Beiboer SH, Wieringa-Jelsma T, Maaskant-Van Wijk PA, et al. Rapid genotyping of blood group antigens by multiplex polymerase chain reaction and DNA microarray hybridization. Transfusion 2005;45:667–79.
23. Denomme GA, Van Oene M. High-throughput multiplex single-nucleotide polymorphism analysis for red cell and platelet antigen genotypes. Transfusion 2005;45:660–6.
24. Peterson JA, Gitter ML, Kanack A, et al. New low-frequency platelet glycoprotein polymorphisms associated with neonatal alloimmune thrombocytopenia. Transfusion 2010;50:324–33.
25. Shehata N, Denomme GA, Hannach B, et al. Mass-scale high-throughput multiplex polymerase chain reaction for human platelet antigen single-nucleotide polymorphisms screening of apheresis platelet donors. Transfusion 2011;51: 2028–33.

26. Vassallo RR. Recognition and management of antibodies to human platelet antigens in platelet transfusion-refractory patients. Immunohematology 2009;25: 119–24.
27. Goldshtein H, Hausmann MJ, Douvdevani A. A rapid direct fluorescent assay for cell-free DNA quantification in biological fluids. Ann Clin Biochem 2009;46: 488–94.
28. Chiu RW, Lo YM. Clinical applications of maternal plasma fetal DNA analysis: translating the fruits of 15 years of research. Clin Chem Lab Med 2013;51: 197–204.
29. Brojer E, Zupanska B, Guz K, et al. Noninvasive determination of fetal RHD status by examination of cell-free DNA in maternal plasma. Transfusion 2005;45: 1473–80.
30. Van der Schoot CE, Soussan AA, Koelewijn J, et al. Non-invasive antenatal RHD typing. Transfus Clin Biol 2006;13:53–7.
31. Cardo L, García BP, Alvarez FV. Non-invasive fetal RHD genotyping in the first trimester of pregnancy. Clin Chem Lab Med 2010;48:1121–6.
32. Scheffer PG, van der Schoot CE, Page-Christiaens GC, et al. Noninvasive fetal blood group genotyping of rhesus D, c, E and of K in alloimmunised pregnant women: evaluation of a 7-year clinical experience. BJOG 2011;118:1340–8.
33. Scheffer PG, Ait Soussan A, Verhagen OJ, et al. Noninvasive fetal genotyping of human platelet antigen-1a. BJOG 2011;118:1392–5.
34. Le Toriellec E, Chenet C, Kaplan C. Safe fetal platelet genotyping: new developments. Transfusion 2013;53(8):1755–62.

Molecular Diagnosis of Hematopoietic Neoplasms

Radhakrishnan Ramchandren, MD[a], Tarek Jazaerly, MD[b],
Ali M. Gabali, MD, PhD[b],*

KEYWORDS

- Hematopoietic neoplasms • Molecular testing • Cytogenetic testing
- Genetic aberrations

KEY POINTS

- Cytogenetic abnormalities are considered to be common events in hematologic malignancies.
- These abnormalities generally consist of structural chromosomal abnormalities or gene mutations, which often are integral to the pathogenesis and subsequent evolution of an individual malignancy.
- Improvements made in identifying and interpreting these molecular alterations has resulted in advances in the diagnosis, prognosis, monitoring, and therapy for cancer.
- As a consequence of the increasingly important role of molecular testing in hematologic malignancy management, we present an update on the importance and use of molecular tests detailing the advantages and disadvantages of each test when applicable.

INTRODUCTION

Hematologic malignancies are associated with diverse genetic aberrations that range from single base-pair substitution to whole chromosomal abnormalities. Before the development of current molecular and cytogenetic techniques, distinguishing between specific diseases was often time consuming and difficult. In the molecular era, however, cytogenetic and molecular tests are commonplace and critical to diagnose hematologic malignancies. Moreover, such testing also plays a significant role in

Conflict of Interest: The authors of this article are acknowledging full responsibility for the work and are not intending to discuss off label or research use of a drug or device. They have no potential conflicts of interest and no significant financial relationship with commercial organizations.
[a] Department of Hematology/Oncology, Karmanos Cancer Institute, Detroit Medical Center, Wayne State University, 3990 John R, Detroit, MI 48201, USA; [b] Department of Pathology, Karmanos Cancer Institute, Detroit Medical Center, Wayne State University, 3990 John R, Detroit, MI 48201, USA
* Corresponding author.
E-mail address: agabal@med.wayne.edu

Clin Lab Med 33 (2013) 817–833
http://dx.doi.org/10.1016/j.cll.2013.08.005
0272-2712/13/$ – see front matter © 2013 Elsevier Inc. All rights reserved.

labmed.theclinics.com

determining prognosis, therapy, and disease status (remission or relapse). The 2008 edition of the World Health Organization (WHO) *Classification of Tumors of Haematopoietic and Lymphoid Tissues* incorporates many new categories of diseases based on molecular signatures.[1] These signatures have the potential to improve the understanding of the disease process and may lead to clinical advances.

MOLECULAR TESTS USED TO IDENTIFY CLONAL T- AND B-CELL POPULATIONS
Immunoglobulin Gene Rearrangement

Immunoglobulins are B-cell receptors (BCR) found on B lymphocytes and able to bind antigens with high specificity. At the protein level, each immunoglobulin (antibody) is formed of heavy chains and light chains. Based on size and amino acid composition, the heavy chains are divided into five isotypes (classes) represented by the Greek letters α, δ, ϵ, γ, and μ, which are representative of the immunoglobulins (Ig) class of heavy chains, IgA, IgD, IgE, IgG, and IgM, respectively. The light chain is much smaller than the heavy chain and consists of one of two possible isotypes, kappa or lambda, that are represented by the Greek letters κ and λ, respectively. The Ig contains two identical heavy chains and two identical light chains. Each chain contains one constant region that is similar for each isotype and one variable region that is different in amino acid sequence for the same isotype. The variable regions of the heavy and light chains undergo gene rearrangement during B-cell development and maturation. An individual B cell, therefore, produces one distinct Ig composed of one unique variable region for the heavy chain and another unique variable region for the light chain.

Humans inherit many variable region gene segments called germline genes. The immunoglobulin heavy chain gene locus (IGH@) is located on chromosome 14q32. However, genes that encode light chains are located on two separate chromosomes. Immunoglobulin kappa locus (IGK@) is located on chromosome 2p11.2 and immunoglobulin lambda locus (IGL@) is located on chromosome 22q11.22. The variable region of the IGH@ contains variable numbers of Variable (V), Diverse (D), and Joining (J) gene regions. The light chains also contain a different number of V and J gene regions, but lack the D gene region.[2,3] These genes are vital for generating the diverse number of human antibodies required and encode for more than 100 variable regions that encode for the first 90 to 95 amino acid of the variable region. The rest of the variable region, the last 15 to 20 amino acids, are present further along the chromosome in a linked set of DNA. Chronologically, the heavy chain variable region rearrangement precedes that of the light chain. Successful IGH rearrangement triggers the rearrangement of IGK@ and failure to achieve successful IGK rearrangement subsequently triggers the rearrangement of IGL@. In addition, the recombination of an individual variable region also occurs in an ordered sequence. The heavy chain recombination first occurs between one randomly selected D and J gene region followed by the joining of one V gene region. Then the constant chain gene is added and similarly the rearrangements of IGK@ and IGL@ start by joining the V and J gene regions to give a VJ complex before the addition of the constant chain gene.[2,3]

T-Cell Gene Rearrangement

Each T-cell receptor (TCR) consists of two different chains coupled together. TCRα (TCRA) and TCRβ (TCRB) chains are present in approximately 95% of the TCR with the rest formed by TCRγ (TCRG) and TCRδ (TCRD) chains. The genes encoding the TCRδ chain are located within the TCRα gene on chromosome 14q11–12, whereas the TCRβ and TCRγ genes are located on chromosome 7q32–35 and 7p15, respectively. Each chain consists of one V and one constant (C) region.[4] The variable coding regions of TCRα and TCRγ are generated by the recombination of VJ regions (like Ig light chain), whereas those that form TCRβ and TCRδ are generated by the recombination of VDJ regions (like Ig heavy chain). The TCR contains different numbers of V, D, and J gene regions. The recombination occurs in a similar pattern to that of immunoglobulin heavy and light chains. Because TCRδ genes are located within the TCRα genes, the rearrangement of TCRα, which occurs first, causes the deletion of the embedded TCRδ gene region.[4]

The basic concept behind testing for immunoglobulin and TCR gene rearrangement is that large numbers of B and/or T cells respond to any single antigen encountered and this leads to having many B and T cells each with different rearranged nongermline variable regions. Neoplastic T and B cells have the same rearranged variable region of the TCR or heavy chain and of the light chain. Most T- and B-cell neoplasms have clonal rearrangement of the variable region that can be detected by various methods including the Southern blot hybridization assay and polymerase chain reaction (PCR) assay.

Southern Blot Analysis for Rearrangement of Immunoglobulin and TCR

Southern blot hybridization is the gold standard assay. The principle of the test is to collect large amounts of DNA material from the tissue of interest; digest it using specific restriction enzymes; and then look for a specific clonal, nongermline pattern. A positive control, usually a cell line, and a negative control, such as water, are also used to compare the results. The digested DNA is run on a gel to separate DNA fragments and then transferred to nitrocellulose membrane. The DNA fragments are visualized by probe hybridization linked to a radioactive material, chromogenic dye or fluorescent dye. For the reasons listed in **Table 1**, currently Southern blot analysis is losing the battle to the PCR assay. One great advantage of Southern blot over PCR is the low false-positive and false-negative results caused by underdigestion and by the presence of polymorphic restriction sites.

PCR Assay for Rearrangement of Immunoglobulin and TCRs

The most targeted region for B-cell neoplasm is the immunoglobulin heavy chain gene; and for the T-cell neoplasm the TCRγ gene region. Accurate knowledge of the rearranged gene segments is required to design primers, and this problem is solved by

Table 1
Technical comparison between Southern blot analysis and PCR assay

Parameter	Southern Blot	PCR Assay
Labor-intensive	Yes	No
Turnaround time	About 7 d	About 3 d
Type of tissue	Fresh tissue	Fresh and fixed paraffin-embedded tissue
Quality of DNA required	Requires 10–20 μg of high-quality DNA	Requires 1–5 μg of DNA
Probe used	Radiolabelled probe gives best results and multiple probes are needed	No radiolabelled probe is used
Sensitivity	Limited sensitivity (5%–10%)	High sensitivity (1%–5%)

the commercial availability of many tested probes with great specificity. In B-cell neoplasm, most PCR probes target the consensus sequence of the J region and the framework segment of the V region of the heavy chain. For many years the drawback of PCR assay of these regions was the false-negative results, especially in tumors that undergo somatic hypermutation and subsequently change the primer binding site.

Diffuse large B-cell lymphoma (DLBCL), follicular lymphoma, subset of chronic lymphocytic leukemia/small lymphocytic lymphoma, and marginal zone lymphoma tend to undergo somatic hypermutation more than others, and the use of additional primers may decrease the false-negative rate in such lesions.[5] Recently, most diagnostic laboratories are using the newly described BIOMED-2 protocol.[6] The assay targets multiple variable gene segments in rearranged immunoglobulin and TCR genes. The primers are designed to probe three VH-JH regions, two DH-JH regions, two IGK regions, one IGL region, three TCRβ regions, two TCRγ regions, and one TCRδ region. This protocol detects almost all clonal B-cell populations including those with a high rate of somatic hypermutation.

In addition, because TCRγ region is rearranged in almost all T-cell neoplasms and many show TCRB gene rearrangements, BIOMED-2 protocol has the ability to detect virtually all clonal T-cell populations.[6,7] However, small clonal B- and T-cell populations have the potential to be missed. On the other hand, because of the high sensitivity of PCR assay, a small number of polyclonal B or T cells could be amplified and cause errorness interpretation of the presence of a clonal population. Therefore, correlation with the morphologic and immunophenotypic findings is required at all times.

OTHER MOLECULAR TESTS USED IN NON-HODGKIN B- AND T-CELL LYMPHOMAS
BCL-2 Translocation Assay

B-cell leukemia/lymphoma-2 (BCL-2) is located on chromosome 18q21.33 and is normally expressed by mantle zone B cells. Immunohistochemical studies demonstrate that primary follicles composed predominantly of B cells are usually positive for BCL-2.[8] T cells also express BCL-2, particularly interfollicular T cells. Germinal center B cells are negative for BCL-2, and positive results may indicate a lymphoma. Follicular lymphoma is the most common lymphoma to express BCL-2 (approximately 85%–90%), and around 20% to 30% of DLBCLs are positive for BCL-2. In lymphomas, BCL-2 protein is abnormal, and results from translocation between chromosome 14 and 18: t(14;18). The placement of the antiapoptotic gene BCL-2 in close proximity to the highly active immunoglobulin gene of the heavy chain causes excessive upregulation of this protein and this potentiates its antiapoptotic activity.

The 2008 edition of the WHO *Classification of Tumors of Haematopoietic and Lymphoid Tissues* incorporates a new provisional category of B-cell neoplasms with features intermediate between DLBCL and Burkitt lymphoma (BL). This entity is characterized by simultaneous t(8;14) and t(14;18) translocations ("double-hit" lymphomas). Studies reported that around 65% of the breakpoints are located at the major breakpoint region (MBR) and around 9% are located at the minor cluster region. The rest of the breakpoints with documented BCL-2 translocation could not be mapped. However, survival studies did not show any correlation between breakpoint location and clinical outcome. The joining (JH6) segment of the immunoglobulin heavy chain was the most frequently involved whatever the breakpoint location. Most primers used in PCR assays target the MBR of BCL-2 and JH6 region of the immunoglobulin heavy chain.

Fluorescence in situ hybridization (FISH) is more sensitive in detecting BCL-2 translocation than PCR assay. This is because PCR assay is limited by the size of the primer needed for the PCR reaction, whereas FISH can use large spanning probes, because all that is needed is hybridization of the probe to its complimentary sequence. Studies found that the higher the grade of follicular lymphoma the more likely it is *not* to show BCL-2 translocation. As with all ancillary tests, correlation with the morphologic findings is required, because low levels of BCL-2 can be detected in the peripheral blood of normal individuals.

Cyclin-D1 Translocation Assay

Cyclin-D 1 (CCND1), also known as BCL-1, is located on chromosome 11q13.3 and is the hallmark of mantle cell lymphoma (MCL). CCND1 is also expressed by a subset of plasma cell myeloma. CCND1-positive myeloma is also positive for t(11;14), and most myeloma cells are CD20 positive with the morphologic appearance of small plasmcytoid lymphocytes. In addition, a small subset of hairy cell leukemia may show weak expression of CCND1 protein, but they are predominantly negative for t(11;14). The t(11;14) places CCND1 gene in juxtaposition to the highly active immunoglobulin gene of the heavy chain causing overexpression of CCND1 protein. CCND1 is a nuclear, cell-cycle control protein and in normal cells is maximally expressed in G1 phase.[9] All normal lymphocytes are negative for CCND1 expression by immunohistochemical studies.

In approximately 50% of MCL, the breakpoint of the translocation is located at one area termed major translocation cluster. However, the rest of the breakpoints are not linked to any specific region. Therefore, the PCR assay is not that sensitive for CCND1 translocation. FISH analysis using large, dual-fusion probes is the most sensitive assay. Less than 5% of classic cases of MCLs are CCND1-negative. The diagnosis of such category becomes more difficult because this lymphoma is usually negative for t(11;14). Identification of SOX11 protein in neoplastic cells may be helpful in such a scenario.[10]

BCL-6 Translocation Assay

BCL-6 is a transcriptional repressor that blocks the maturation of B cells to plasma cells and is essential for the formation of germinal centers.[11] The BCL6 gene is located on chromosome 3q27.3, and the protein is normally expressed in the nuclei of germinal center B and T cells. The 3q27 translocation affecting BCL-6 gene has been observed in 20% to 40% of DLBCL and in 5% to 10% of follicular lymphoma. The partner of a BCL-6 translocated gene can be an Ig or non-Ig partner. In one study, a total of 120 BCL-6 breakpoint found that 62 breakpoints (52%) joined to immunoglobulin heavy chain; 12 to immunoglobulin light chains (10%); and 46 to non-Ig partners (38%). Around 20 non-Ig partner genes have been identified, including 1p32, 7p11, 7p21, 14q11, and 16p13. Some studies suggest that DLBCL with non-Ig/BCL-6 fusion has a poor prognosis. Breakpoints at 3q27 are predominantly located in the 5′ untranslated region of BCL6 that has been called the MBR.[12] As with BCL-2, many of the breakpoints may locate outside the MBR. Thus, the PCR assay using specific probes may not detect BCL-6 rearrangement. Many diagnostic laboratories are using FISH break-apart probes spanning the BCL6 locus and not the dual fusion IGH@/BCL6-specific probes.

Cellular Myelocytomatosis Translocation Assay

Cellular myelocytomatosis (C-MYC) gene is a transcription factor located on chromosome 8q24. In normally growing cells, C-MYC is produced in small amounts. This production is tightly regulated during cell cycle and it returns back to its basal level in nondividing cells. Abnormally produced C-MYC activates a protective pathway through the induction of p53-dependent cell death pathway, among others, such as p14ARF and BCL-2 like protein11 (BIM), which forces such cells to undergo apoptosis. p53 plays an important role in MYC-induced apoptosis, and around 30% of endemic BL harbor a p53 mutation. BL is characterized by having C-MYC translocation with the JH region of immunoglobulin heavy chain (14q32) (80%) and less frequently with the loci of immunoglobulin light chains (kappa or lambda), with slight preference for partnering with kappa (15%) than lambda (5%) gene segments.

C-MYC is detected in virtually all cases of BL and in high numbers of AIDS-related lymphoma including Epstein-Barr virus–positive and Epstein-Barr virus–negative cases. C-MYC detection plays a major role in diagnosing the new provisional WHO 2008 entity of B-cell lymphoma with features intermediate between DLBCL and BL, as discussed previously. In the latter, the C-MYC partner is usually nonimmunoglobulin associated. In addition to being reported in de novo cases of DLBCL (10%), some cases of Richter transformation of chronic lymphocytic leukemia/small lymphocytic lymphoma have C-MYC translocation.[13] C-MYC is also detected in other lymphomas and plasma cell myeloma with much less frequency.

Based on the chromosomal breakpoints relative to the C-MYC gene, the translocations have been classified into three classes. Translocations within the 5′ first noncoding exon or intron of 5′ region of C-MYC gene have been designated as class I, those with breakpoints immediately upstream of the gene as class II, and those with breakpoints distant as class III. Studies have found that the breakpoints in BL are different between the sporadic and endemic entities of BL. All cases of BL have C-MYC translocation; however, rearrangement of C-MYC gene, close to the 5′ first noncoding exon or intron region, is predominantly demonstrated in sporadic BL (class I). C-MYC gene in most cases of endemic BL is translocated as an intact nonrearranged gene. In this case the breakpoint in chromosome 8 is found to be outside the C-MYC gene (class III).

Several methods are used to detect C-MYC translocation including conventional cytogenetics (CCs), Southern blot, and FISH. Among all, FISH detection is the method most used by laboratories. Because C-MYC translocations show no constant clustering of breakpoints, the PCR detection method is not the best test to look for C-MYC translocation. Both fusion and break-apart probes are used. Break-apart probes, designed to span most of the C-MYC region, are usually applied to test for C-MYC rearrangement including those arising from variant translocations. Specific fusion probes are then applied to detect the t(8;14), t(2;8), and t(8;22) abnormalities. However, up to 10% of BL cases may lack a demonstrable C-MYC translocation by FISH. In this case Southern blot hybridization probes hybridizing to class II and class III region may be helpful to detect translocations in such cases.

Mucosal-associated Lymphoid Tissue Translocation Assay

The t(11;18)(q21;q21) is the most common translocation in mucosal-associated lymphoid tissue (MALT) lymphomas and is found in approximately 30% to 40% of MALT lymphoma. The next encountered translocation is t(14;18) (q32;q21), which is seen in around 10% to 20% of cases.[14,15] The most common sites for the t(11;18)(q21;q21) are stomach and lung, and it involves the gene of API2, member of the apoptosis suppressor family on chromosome 11q21 and MALT1 gene on chromosome 18q21. The t(14;18) involves the immunoglobulin heavy chain locus 14q32 and the MALT gene 18q21 and is detected in MALT lymphoma of the liver, skin, ocular adnexa, and salivary glands but less frequently in MALT lymphoma involving other sites.

Other translocations have been described in MALT lymphoma including t(1;14)/IGH-BCL10 and t(3;14)/IGH-FOXP1. The last two translocations are rare, found in around 2% of MALT lymphoma each and they are not confined to any specific site. Continuous activation of nuclear factor kappa B is the main mechanism by which the t(11;18)/API2-MALT1, t(14;18)/IGH-MALT1, and t(1;14)/IGH-BCL10 promote lymphoma. The function of the t(3;14)/IGH-FOXP1 in MALT lymphoma remains unclear.

Gastric lymphomas with t(11;18)/API2-MALT1 respond poorly to treatment directed against *Helicobacter pylori* microorganism. They show less than 10% of durable remission at long-term follow-up, and they may spread to regional lymph nodes or distal sites. However, most high-grade transformation of MALT lymphomas is seen in nontranslocation-associated lymphoma rather than those with positive translocation. Interestingly, neoplastic cells of MALT lymphoma associated with either t(11;18) or t(1;14) demonstrate nuclear expression of BCL-10 by immunohistochemistry.

As with other low-grade lymphomas, using CC analysis for detecting MALT translocations is hampered by the low yield and poor quality of metaphase spreads. In addition, cytogenetic analysis cannot differentiate between t(14;18) caused by IGH/BCL-2 and that caused by IGH/MALT1 because the 18q21 region contains the BCL-2 and MALT1 loci. Therefore, interphase FISH is becoming the main test to look for such translocations.

Anaplastic Lymphoma Kinase Translocation Assay

Anaplastic lymphoma kinase (ALK, CD246) is a type II transmembrane receptor tyrosine kinase and is a member of the insulin receptor superfamily involved in the development of the nervous system. ALK is not expressed in normal and hyperplastic lymphoid tissue. Approximately 85% of pediatric and 35% of adult anaplastic large cell lymphoma (ALCL) is associated with a recurrent cytogenetic abnormality that involves ALK in locus 2p23.[16] ALK protein is also expressed by a subset of DLBCL. Deregulated ALK fusion protein has been reported in neural origin tumors, such as retinoblastoma and neuroblastoma, and some cases of lung carcinoma and melanoma.

In ALCL, ALK expression is associated with better 5-year survival rates when compared with ALK-negative ALCL. The most common partner for ALK protein is the nucleophosmin (NPM) gene located at 5q35 and is seen in around 80% of the ALK-positive ALCL. NPM is a nucleolar protein responsible for protein shuttling between the cytoplasm and the nucleus. The t(2;5) results in expression of a novel fusion protein, NPM-ALK (also called p80) that has tyrosine kinase activity and has been shown to induce a lymphoma-like disease in mice. By immunohistochemistry, the NPM-ALK fusion protein can be nuclear or cytoplasmic.

Other partner genes have been described in about 15% to 20% of ALK-positive ALCL including TRK fused gene (TFG) at 3q21, TFG-ALK, tropomysin 3 (TPM3) at locus 1q25, topomysin 4 (TPM4) at locus 19p13, and clathrin chain polypeptide-like gene at locus 17q11 among others.[17] No difference in survival is seen between the ALK-NPM translocation and the variant translocations. When ALK partners with other than NPM gene, it produces cytoplasmic or membranous staining patterns by immunohistochemical studies.

NPM-ALK fusion transcripts can be detected by PCR using primers targeting the ALK portion of the transcript. However, because low levels of detection can be seen in the peripheral blood and lymph node of healthy individuals, only the high-level detection matches with the presence of ALK fusion gene identified by CCs and FISH studies. In most laboratories, the FISH break-apart probes that hybridize to the two ends of the ALK gene breakpoint are routinely used to detect the t(2;5) and variant translocations, because documenting ALK translocation is more clinically important than identifying its partner chromosome.

MOLECULAR TESTS USED TO IDENTIFY DEFINING CYTOGENETIC ABNORMALITIES OF THE LEUKEMIAS
Acute Myeloid Leukemia with t(15;17)(q22;q21)/PML-RARA

In acute myeloid leukemia (AML) the identification of t(15;17)(q22;q21) is diagnostic of acute promyelocytic leukemia (APL), representing approximately 10% of AML. In addition to having this defining cytogenetic abnormality, APL has its own distinctive morphologic and immunophenotypic characteristics with high prediction of the disease. The urgency of early diagnosis of APL is generally attributed to a tendency to develop disseminated intravascular coagulation and the responsiveness of the disease to all-*trans* retinoic acid (ATRA) and arsenic trioxide therapy. The presence of t(15;17), and t(8;21) and inv(16), as a solo abnormality in AML is associated with a favorable prognosis.

The t(15;17)(q22;q21) involves the promyelocytic leukemia (PML) gene from chromosome 15 and the retinoic acid receptor-alpha (RARA) gene from chromosome 17 to produce PML-RARA fusion gene or RARA-PML reciprocal product. In most cases, the breakpoint on chromosome 17 is located in intron 2 of the RARA gene. However, the PML gene has three breakpoint cluster regions (bcr) called bcr1 at intron 6 (long, L-form), bcr2 at exon 6 (variant, V-form), and bcr3 at intron 6 (short, S-form) forms based on the size of the end products. The L- and S-forms represent approximately 90% of the t(15;17) positive cases.

Generally, the t(15;17) can be detected in 98% of typical APL cases. The rest (2%) of typical APL cases have either a cryptic (submicroscopic) PML breakpoint or RARA translocation with rare variants, including t(11;17)(q23;q21) that forms the PML zinc-finger protein-RARA fusion (PLZF-RARA), t(5;17)(q35;q21) that forms NPM-RARA fusion, t(11;17)(q13;q21) that generates nuclear mitotic apparatus-RARA transcript (NUMA-RARA), and der(17) that forms the signal transducer and activator of transcription-RARA fusion (STAT5b-RARA).[18,19] Few other variants have been reported to partner with the RARA gene; however, their novelty has to be confirmed. Variants PLZF-RARA and NPM-RARA fusion genes may have reciprocal products. Patients with APL with PLZF-RARA gene fusion may respond to histone deacetylase inhibitors rather than ATRA or arsenic trioxide therapy.

Peripheral blood or bone marrow samples can be used to look for the t(15;17) or other variant translocation abnormalities. CC may detect 75% of the APL associated translocations. However, the major problem with CC is the increased risk of false-negatives. FISH is considered more sensitive, and it can detect up to 98% of the cases when the correct probes are used. Both dual-color fusion probes and break-apart probes can be used, even though the latter needs further work-up. In cases with cryptic PML fusion gene, or when minimal residual disease is to be investigated, FISH analysis on different metaphases and interphases from cytogenetic cultures has been shown to be useful. Reverse transcriptase (RT)-PCR also can be used in such conditions. The only caveat is that sometimes RT-PCR may produce several bands in patient sample with bcr2 PML breakpoint, and they could be potentially misinterpreted as nonspecific amplification products.

AML with t(8;21)(q22;q22)/RUNX1-RUNX1T1

The t(8;21) constitutes approximately 5% to 10% of all cases of AML and it results from the fusion of Runt-related transcription factor 1 (RUNX1) gene on 21q22 and the RUNX1T1 (RUNX1- translocated to 1) gene on 8q22.[20] RUNX1, also known as AML 1 protein (AML1) and core-binding factor subunit alpha-2 (CBFA2), is expressed by all hematopoietic elements. Core binding factor includes the DNA binding unite RUNX1 (in addition to RUNX2 and RUNX3 subunits) and the non-DNA binding CBF subunit-Beta (CBFB). All four subunits are necessary for the formation of normal hematopoietic stem cells during embryogenesis. RUNX1T1, also known as Eight Twenty One, is a transcription regulatory protein that binds to nuclear histone deacetylases and transcription factors to block differentiation of hematopoietic elements. Some reports indicate that around 3% of AML associated with t(8;21) have variant translocations for which their significance needs to be clarified. The breakpoint in both genes of RUNX1 and RUNX1T1 are clustered in highly conserved regions, intron 5-6 in RUNX1and in intron 1b-2 in RUNX1T1. Therefore, most of the translocations create a fusion transcript made of the 5' region of RUNX1 fused to the 3' region of RUNX1T1 gene and form the same fusion transcript that can be detected in all patients. The t(8;21) can be detected by CC and FISH analysis using locus-specific probes for AML1–Eight Twenty One fusion. False-negative results in FISH analysis may occur if the malignant cells represent less than 10% of the cells present in the specimen. In such situations RT-PCR analyses can also be used to detect and confirm the presence of the RUNX1-RUNX1T1 fusion gene.

AML with inv(16)(p13.1q22) or t(16;16)(p13.1;q22)/CBFB-MYH11

The inv(16) and t(16;16) occur in around 5% of pediatric and 7% of adult AML cases. However, most cases of AML with abnormal eosinophils (AML-M4Eo) are associated with inv(16)(p13.1q22) or, to a lesser extent, with t(16;16)(p13.1;q22).[21] Both result in the fusion of the CBFB gene at 16q22 to the myosin heavy chain 11 (MYH11) gene at 16p13.1 locus. Even though the CBFB–MYH11 chimeric protein tends to be sequestered in the cytoplasm, it has the ability to interfere with the function, in a dominant-negative manner, of CBF. Such mechanism is postulated to impair cell differentiation and increase predisposion to leukemic cell transformation. The breakpoint in CBFB gene occurs in intron 5, but the breakpoint in MYH11 is variable and includes more than 8 regions on the gene. Therefore, CC analysis may overlook cryptic (submicroscopic) fusion. In such condition, the use of FISH and RT-PCR methods may be important to detect CBFB/MYH11 fusion gene. Other structural abnormalities are seen in around 30% to 40% of cases including trisomy 22, trisomy 8, and 7q deletion. Because trisomy 22 is rare in other acute leukemias, the presence of trisomy 22 without detectable inv(16) or t(16;16) by CC may suggest the presence of a possible cryptic genetic alteration.

Acute Leukemia with 11q23/Mixed Lineage Leukemia Translocation

Mixed lineage leukemia (MLL) gene is located at 11q23 locus and it functions as a positive regulatory gene in hematopoiesis development during embryogenesis.[22] The presence of rearranged MLL gene is considered an unfavorable prognostic indicator and is observed in approximately 3% to 4% of AML and in around 3% to 7% of acute lymphoblastic leukemia (ALL). In fact, translocated MLL gene is seen in AML and ALL affecting adult and infant patients, and in most patients with therapy-related acute leukemia caused by previous history of topoisomerase II inhibitor therapy.[22] Breakpoints in the MLL gene are located between exon 5 and 11. To date, more than 100 translocations have been reported to partner with the MLL gene and most of them are cloned. Three partners have been identified in around 80% including AF4 (ALL-1 fused gene on chromosome 4) gene to form t(4;11)(q21;q23); MLLT3 (myeloid/lymphoid mixed lineage leukemia translocate 3) gene to create t(9;11)(q21;q23); and MLLT1 gene to form t(11;19)(q23;p13). Rearrangement of 11q23 can be detected by CC, FISH analysis, and other molecular tests including Southern blot hybridization and RT-PCR. The CC ability to detect such rearrangement is limited by the presence of cryptic fusion particularly when its partner has a telomeric location. FISH is useful in such circumstances. In addition, FISH can discriminate between true 11q23/MLL and rearrangements clustering within the 11q22 to 25 regions without MLL involvement. RT-PCR is the most sensitive approach for detecting specific subtypes of MLL rearrangements when the partner gene is known, otherwise multiplex RT-PCR approach is used.

ACUTE LEUKEMIA WITH OTHER TRANSLOCATIONS
AML with t(6;9)(p23;q34)/DEK-NUP214

This translocation is seen in approximately 1% to 2% of acute leukemia affecting children and adults. The DEK-NUP214 chimeric protein encodes for altered nucleoporin fusion protein with an aberrant transcription factor activity that affects nuclear transport. This translocation is associated with poor prognosis, multilineage dysplasia, basophilia, and higher association with FLT3-ITD mutation. Some reports indicate the presence of terminal deoxynucleotidyl transferase (TdT) in neoplastic cells. The breakpoints in both genes are constant and this allows for the design of specific probe for precise detection by RT-PCR.

AML with inv(3)(q21q26.2) or t(3;3)(q21;q26.2)/RPN1-EVI1

This translocation is seen in 1% to 2% of adult AML and is associated with poor response to therapy and dismal outcome. It results in the juxtaposition of the ribophorin 1(RPN1) gene with the ecotropic viral integration site-1 (EVI1) gene that causes defective cellular proliferation and differentiation, and subsequent leukemic transformation. Inv(3) AML is associated with multilineage dysplasia with atypical megakaryocytes, variable fibrosis, and peripheral thrombocytosis.[23] Secondary cytogenetic abnormalities are seen in about 40% of cases including monosomy 7, 5q del, and complex karyotypes. Rearrangement of EVI1 gene at 3q26 locus with other chromosomes including t(1;3)(p36.3;q21.1) and t(3;21)(q26.2;q22.1), t(2;3)(p15;q26.2), and t(3;12)(q26.2;p13) are excluded. The former two translocations are commonly seen in AML with myelodysplasia-related changes. The chromosomal breakpoints at 3q26 in the translocation are in the 5′ of the EVI1 gene, whereas the breakpoints in the inversion cases are at the 3′ of the gene. The fusion transcript can be detected by RT-PCR and FISH analysis using dual-color probes, now commercially available.

AML (Megakaryoblastic) with t(1;22)(p13;q13)/RBM15-MKL1

This translocation is restricted to patients younger than 3 years old and constitutes approximately 1% of AML. Morphologically, it is linked to acute megakaryoblastic leukemia and commonly associated with variable amounts of bone marrow fibrosis, hepatosplenomegaly, and poor outcome. The translocation results in the fusion of RNA-binding motif protein 15 (RBM15) and megakaryocyte leukemia 1 genes (MKL1). It has been postulated that the fusion protein causes impairment of megakaryoblastic proliferation and differentiation.

The t(1;22) can be detected by CC or FISH analysis. Some laboratories are using RT-PCR to identify the chimeric mRNA.

ACUTE LEUKEMIA WITH GENE MUTATIONS
NPM1 Mutated AML

NPM1 mutations occur in about 50% of normal karyotypes of AML and about 35% in AML associated with chromosomal aberration.[24,25] Physiologically, NPM1 is a nucleolar protein that mediates the transport of ribosomal proteins through the nuclear membrane. Aberration affecting NPM1 causes its sequestration in the cytoplasm, thus preventing its function as a transport protein. Deregulated NPM1 gene (5q35) may result from balanced translocation (t(2;5)(p23;q35)/ALK-NPM1, t(5;17)(q35;q21)/NPM-RARA, and t(3;5)(q25.1;q34)/MLF1-NPM1) or mutation.

The most common mutation is an insertion of four-base pairs, in exon 12, resulting in a frame-shift and replacement of the seven C-terminal amino acids of the NPM1 protein by 11 different residues that causes the disruption of the nucleolar localization signal. Some studies indicated that mutated NPM1 inhibits the tumor-suppressor gene p14-ARF. NPM1 mutations often coincide with mutations in FLT3 and such association may decrease its favorable outcome. NPM1 mutation is analyzed by PCR amplification followed by fragment analysis by capillary electrophoresis to detect small insertional mutations.

CCAAT Enhancer Binding Protein Alpha Mutated AML

CCAAT enhancer binding protein alpha is a transcription factor that is involved in myeloid cell differentiation. Mutated CCAAT enhancer binding protein alpha is found in around 10% of AML and is associated with good prognosis. Mutations may involve both alleles with one allele having mutation in C-terminus and the other allele in N-terminus.[24,25] Less frequently, one allele with both C and N-termini mutations may present. Mutations are detected by PCR amplification followed by sequencing.

Fms-related Tyrosine Kinase 3 Gene Mutated AML

Fms-related tyrosine kinase 3 gene (FLT3) is a tyrosine kinase receptor that is involved in cell maturation and inhibition of apoptosis. Mutated FLT3 is found in approximately 30% of AML and is associated with poor outcome.[24,25] FLT3 may undergo point mutation of the aspartic acid residue 835 (D835) on exon 20 or internal tandem duplication (ITD) of the juxtamembrane domain on exon 14/15. FLT3 mutations are detected by multiplex PCR amplification followed by capillary electrophoresis for length mutations (FLT3-ITD) and resistance to EcoRV digestion (D835). Studies have found that high mutant/wild-type ratio is associated with worse prognosis.

KIT Mutated Leukemia

cKIT (CD117) is the cellular homolog of the feline sarcoma viral oncogene v-kit. It is a class III receptor tyrosine kinase that is involved in stem cell homing to their microenvironment, and the gene is located at 4q11-q12.[24,25] cKIT mutations are gain of function mutations, and they result from an ITD of exon 11 or insertion/deletion of exon 8 at the tyrosine kinase domain. The presence of cKIT mutation, particularly in the setting of core binding leukemia (t[8;21] and inv[16]), is associated with poor outcome. cKIT mutations are detected by using allele-specific PCR and sequencing.

Wilms' Tumor Gene Mutated Leukemia

Wilms' tumor gene (WT1) is a transcription factor that has tumor suppressor and, paradoxically, oncogenic functions. The gene is located at 11p13 and most mutations are present on exons 7 and 9.[24,25] It is seen in about 10% to 14% of AML and its expression is associated with poor prognosis. WT1 mutations are detected by using allele-specific PCR followed by amplicon sequencing and computer analysis for the presence of mutation.

Leukemia Associated with Isocitrate Dehydrogenase 1 and 2 or "Brain And Acute Leukemia, Cytoplasmic"

Some proteins have been reported to be overexpressed in AML, particularly in AML with normal karyotype, and they may act as adverse prognostic factors.[24] Mutations involving isocitrate dehydrogenase 1 (IDH1, IDH1^{R132}) and 2 (IDH2, IDH2^{R172}) and "the brain and acute leukemia, cytoplasmic" genes are among this group. Basically, they are detected by PCR amplification and mutational analysis by sequencing and comparison with the published unmutated sequence.

ALL with t(9;22)(q34;q11)/BCR-ABL

The t(9;22) translocation is seen in 25% and 5% of adult and pediatric B-ALL, respectively. Almost all cases of chronic myelogenous leukemia (CML) have t(9;22). The translocation involves the fusion of ABL (Abelson murine leukemia viral oncogene homolog 1) gene at 9q34 with BCR (breakpoint cluster region protein) gene at 22q11. Philadelphia (Ph) chromosome is the derivative chromosome 22 and is associated with poor outcome in B-ALL. In CML and ALL the cluster region in ABL gene is somewhat constant, however, depending on the cluster breakpoints (major [M-BCR], minor [m-BCR], and micro [μ-BCR]) in the BCR gene, three fusion transcripts with high tyrosine activities are produced. Breakpoints in the cluster regions M-BCR, m-BCR, and μ-BCR translate into p210, p190, and p230 proteins, respectively. The former is the most common breakpoint in CML (95%). The breakpoint in ALL is in the m-BCR region. This translocation can be detected by several methods including CC, Southern blotting, FISH, and RT-PCR. The latter is the most commonly used test particularly when looking for minimal residual disease.

ALL with t(12;21)(p13;q22)/TEL/RUNX1

This translocation is found in around 20% to 30% and 3% of pediatric and adult B-ALL, respectively, and most of the time in cryptic form. B-ALL with t(12;21) demonstrates favorable prognosis but this observation is hindered by late relapse. The translocation involves fusion of intron 5 of TEL gene at 12p13 locus with intron 1 of RUNX1 gene at 21q22. The mechanism by which this fusion protein works is not completely revealed; however, it seems to interfere with RUNX1-dependent gene regulation. Because of the cryptic nature of this translocation CC analysis is not the preferred test. Both FISH and RT-PCR are used to detect t(12;21).

ALL with t(1;19)(q23;p13)/TCF3-PBX1

This translocation is seen in about 5% of pediatric B-ALL and is associated with poor prognosis. It results from the fusion of T-cell factor 3 (TCF3) gene at 19p13 and the pre–B-cell leukemia transcription factor 1 (PBX1) at 1q23. The chimeric protein causes impairment of B-cell maturation and proliferation. In about 25% of cases the translocation is cryptic, thus precluding its detection by CCs. FISH and RT-PCR can be also used to detect t(1;19).

ALL with t(4;11)(q11;q23)/AF4-MLL

This translocation is seen in approximately 10% of adult and pediatric B-ALL and in about 80% of infantile B-ALL. B-ALL associated with this translocation has poor prognosis in all age groups. It results from the fusion of MLL gene at 11q23 with AF4 gene at 4q11. FISH and RT-PCR can be used to detect this translocation.

CML with t(9;22)(q34;q11)/BCR-ABL1

The discovery of Ph chromosome in 1960 provided the first evidence of a genetic association to cancer. The translocation involves the fusion of ABL gene at 9q34 with the BCR gene at 22q11.[26,27] Ph chromosome is the shortened chromosome number 22 because of this translocation. Ph chromosome harbors the gene that encodes for the chimeric protein BCR-ABL1 that exhibits high kinase activity and results in phosphorylation and recruitment of several cellular substrates. BCR-ABL1 fusion protein induces myeloid proliferation through many pathways including P13K/AKT, JAK/STAT, RAS/RAF, and JUN.[27] Studies show that the reciprocal ABL/BCR on chromosome 9 encodes p96 and p40 fusion proteins. Their leukemogenic potential is under investigation.

Almost all cases of typical CML are positive for t(9;22). The CML cases with negative Ph chromosome by cytogenetic and molecular studies are in the category of myelodysplastic/myeloproliferative neoplasm (MDS/MPN) in the 2008 WHO classification. Further description of the BCR-ABL1 fusion protein is described previously. Imatinib mesylate (Gleevec) has an inhibitory effect on the continuously activated ABL1 domain of the BCR-ABL1 chimeric protein. In addition to imatinib, the new-generation drugs dasatinib and nilotinib have improved the outcome of CML. However, new BCR-ABL1 mutations have been implicated in some resistant cases of CML. Approximately 85% of all resistance-associated mutations are caused by a single amino acid substitution including T315I, F359V, Y253F/H, M244V, G250E, E255K/V, and M351T. The new generation drugs can be used in cases with resistance-associated mutations.

Conventional karyotype can detect the t(9;22), except the cryptic forms (around 5%), where FISH analysis can be used. The advantage of CC over FISH is that it also can reveal additional chromosomal abnormalities that are harbingers of accelerated phase or blast crisis. Most laboratories are using quantitative RT-PCR to measure BCR-ABL1 p210, P230, and p190 transcripts. The quantitative RT-PCR results are normalized to the international standard (IS) and presented in "IS % ratio" units. For example, a sensitivity of 0.001 IS % ratio indicates the detection of 1 translocation positive cell per 100,000 cells.[28]

MUTATIONS ASSOCIATED WITH MPN

MPN are a heterogeneous group of clonal diseases associated with excessive production of mature hematopoietic elements, including BCR-ABL1–positive CML, polycythemia vera (PV), primary myelofibrosis (PMF) essential thrombocythemia (ET), chronic neutrophilic leukemia, chronic eosinophilic leukemia not otherwise specified (CEN, NOS), mastocytosis and myeloproliferative neoplasms unclassifiable (MPN, NOS). Mutations involving Janus kinase 2 (JAK2V617F), myeloproliferative leukemia (MPL) protein, and JAK2 exon 12 cause constitutive activation of cytokine-regulated intracellular signaling pathways, which are considered the major driving mechanism of BCR-ABL1–negative MPN. The 2008 edition of the WHO incorporates JAK2 mutations (V617F and exon 12) in the diagnostic criteria for the diagnosis of PV, PMF, and ET. In JAK2 mutation–negative cases of MPN, the finding of MPL mutation addresses the WHO criteria.

The JAK2 mutations are the most common mutations in MPN where they are identified in most patients with PV (95%), in about half of the patients with PMF or ET, and rarely with other MPN, myelodysplastic syndrome (MDS), and MPN/MDS. JAK2 is a downstream tyrosine kinase involved in the phosphorylation and activation of different cellular proteins, which mediate different cellular functions, including cell growth and differentiation. The gene encoding JAK2 is located at 9p24 locus. The first identified

JAK2 mutation involves a change of valine to phenylalanine at the 617 position in exon 14 (JAK2V617F). Other mutations have been found to occur in the 3' terminus of exon 12 of JAK2 gene (JAK2 exon 12 mutation) in patients with JAK2V617F-negative MPN (1%–5%). JAK2 mutations are gain-of-function mutations causing constitutive activation of tyrosine kinase and subsequent activation of cytokine-regulated intracellular signaling pathways. MPL is another protein that was found to play a role in the pathogenesis of MPN with negative JAK2 mutations. MPL mutations are caused by a substitution of leucine, lysine, or alanine for tryptophan at codon 515 (W515L, W515K, and S505N), and these mutations have been reported in around 5% and 1% of PMF and ET cases, respectively. The presence of MPL mutations is associated with severe anemia and thrombocytosis. JAK2 and MPL mutations are detected by using allele-specific PCR amplification followed by amplicon sequencing for mutation detection. The tests are resulted as positive or negative. The sensitivity of the test is limited by the presence of mutant allele (1%–10%) in the background of wild-type allele. In JAK2V617F-positive cases evaluating melting curve differentiates wild-type (GG) from homozygous (GT) and heterozygous (TT) mutants.

A new category that is incorporated in the 2008 WHO edition is myeloid and lymphoid neoplasms associated with eosinophilia and abnormalities of platelet-derived growth factor (PDGF) receptor alpha (PDGFRA) at 4q12 locus, PDGF receptor beta (PDGFRB) at 5q33 locus, or epidermal growth factor receptor 1 at 8p11.2 locus. These genes encode cell surface tyrosine kinase receptors that regulate embryonic development and cell proliferation and differentiation. Cases associated with rearrangement of PDGFRA and FGFR1 tends to have a lymphoid component and may present initially as T- or B-lymphoblastic leukemia/lymphoma with eosinophilia, whereas cases associated with PDGFRB tend to present as chronic myelomonocytic leukemia with eosinophilia or as CEL. Myeloid neoplasms associated with PDGFRA or PDGFRB rearrangements are sensitive to imatinib (Gleevec) therapy. Rearrangement of PDGFRB and FGFR1 can be detected by CC and by FISH and PCR amplification and sequencing. However, because of the cryptic nature of PDGFRA rearrangement, molecular testing through PCR amplification and sequencing PCR is usually necessary.

CYTOGENETIC ABNORMALITIES ASSOCIATED WITH MDS

MDS is a group of diseases associated with ineffective hematopoiesis, dysplastic changes in bone marrow elements, and peripheral cytopenia. The 2008 WHO edition of MDS includes refractory cytopenia with unilineage dysplasia (refractory anemia, refractory neutropenia, and refractory thrombocytopenia); refractory anemia with ring sideroblasts; refractory cytopenia with multilineage dysplasia; refractory anemia with excess blasts; MDS with isolated del(5q); MDS-unclassifiable; and childhood MDS including the provisional entity refractory cytopenia of childhood. Most cytogenetic abnormalities are either numerical (loss/gain) or, less commonly, unbalanced/balanced chromosomal abnormalities. They are seen in approximately 80% of secondary MDS after chemotherapy or radiotherapy and in around 50% of de novo cases. The most common abnormalities observed in MDS include monosomy 5 (5-) or deletions in the long arm of chromosome 7 (7q-), 7- or 7q-, 13- or 13q-, trisomy 8 (8+), and 20q-.[29] The balanced translocation that may be seen include t(11;16)(q23;p13.3), t(3;21)(q26.2;q22.1), t(1;3)(p36.3;q21.1), t(2;11)(p21;q23), inv(3)(q21q26.2), and t(6;9)(p23;q34). Around 33% and 40% of MDS cases show a single abnormality or are part of a monosomal karyotype, respectively. Complex karyotypes are seen in about 11% of MDS cases. Conventional karyotypes detect most of the chromosomal abnormalities associated with MDS. FISH analysis and spectral karyotyping also can be used; however, they do not show increased sensitivity over CC.

THE IMPORTANCE OF CHROMOSOMAL ABERRATIONS IN HEMATOPOIETIC MALIGNANCIES

It is not surprising that an accurate diagnosis is important in the management of hematopoietic neoplasms. Given the ever-expanding list of diagnostic disorders, an increasing understanding of the molecular biology of cancer, the proliferation of sensitive testing methods, and novel targeted therapies designed to capitalize on these findings, it is also clear this process has never been more difficult or critical for appropriate patient care. Indeed, when coupled with the appropriate clinical scenario, molecular markers have proved to be beneficial and often vital to the diagnosis, prognosis, and therapy for hematologic malignancies.

A prime example of this is detailed in the story of CML. The identification of the t(9;22) translocation resulting in the fusion of BCR and ABL, results in constitutively active fusion tyrosine kinase. The identification of this abnormality by cytogenetics, FISH, or PCR is necessary for the diagnosis of CML. The phenotypic and clinical conditions that mimic CML, such as other myeloproliferative syndromes, leukemoid reactions, and chronic myelomonocytic leukemia, fail to possess this crucial translocation. This critical discrepancy allows physicians to more accurately diagnose CML in the molecular era. More importantly, scientists have developed several tyrosine kinase inhibitors to inhibit the hyperactive fusion protein coded by the (9;22) translocation. These tyrosine kinase inhibitors have transformed a universally fatal illness to one with an excellent prognosis.

Other such examples of molecularly targeted therapies are noted in other hematologic disorders. For instance, the use of ATRA in APL has capitalized on the improved understanding of disease pathophysiology. In APL a translocation of the retinoic acid receptor on chromosome 17 occurs (most commonly with the PML gene on chromosome 15) and the resultant fusion protein inhibits myeloid differentiation. The use of ATRA overcomes this phenomenon and has been used extensively in the treatment of APL.

Other chromosomal abnormalities in AML engender a favorable, intermediate, or unfavorable prognosis and are used in combination with other factors to help determine when allogeneic transplants are considered. In this way the prognostic implications of molecular testing may also result in alteration of management.

Molecular findings also provide potential insights into the underlying pathophysiology of malignancy and help clinicians understand why in some instances treatment is unsuccessful. For instance, the inv(16) chromosomal abnormality in AML is generally associated with a good prognosis with conventional chemotherapy. Studies suggest high rates of complete remission and 10-year survivals of more than 50% in this population with conventional therapy. Several patients with this cytogenetic abnormality fail to remain in remission, however, and studies have suggested that at least a proportion of these failures may be related to mutations in c-kit. In one study approximately 30% of inv(16) patients harbored a c-kit mutation and had higher incidences of relapse and a lower overall survival rate when compared with their wild-type c-kit counterparts. Consequently, because of interactions between individual molecular abnormalities, favorable prognosis leukemia may be altered negatively. Similarly in lymphoma, overexpression of C-MYC and BCL-2 translocations, so called "double-hit lymphomas," have been shown to confer a poorer prognosis to conventional therapy. However, neither C-MYC overexpression, nor presences of the BCL-2 translocation have been shown to result in poorer outcomes, which raises the possibility of important interactions between individual abnormalities.

Lastly, the ability to identify these signatures of malignancy allows for sensitive monitoring of response or relapse. The (9;22) translocation in CML is assessed by PCR to determine the depth of response. This translocation is also commonly seen in ALL and is a sensitive predictor of relapse on completion of therapy.

SUMMARY

The progress made by advances in molecular medicine has had far reaching effects in all aspects of clinical treatment of hematologic malignancies. These findings, and numerous others, have provided a doorway into understanding the molecular drivers of disease but have also yielded excellent targets for therapy, thereby saving numerous lives.

REFERENCES

1. Vardiman JW, Thiele J, Arber DA, et al. The 2008 revision of the World Health Organization (WHO) classification of myeloid neoplasms and acute leukemia: rationale and important changes. Blood 2009;114:937–51.
2. Alt FW, Yancopoulos GD, Blackwell TK, et al. Ordered rearrangement of immunoglobulin heavy chain variable region segments. EMBO J 1984;3:1209–19.
3. Tonegawa S. Somatic generation of antibody diversity. Nature 1983;302:575–81.
4. Davis MM, Bjorkman PJ. T-cell antigen receptor genes and T-cell recognition. Nature 1988;334:395–402.
5. Tobin G, Rosenquist R. Prognostic usage of V(H) gene mutation status and its surrogate markers and the role of antigen selection in chronic lymphocytic leukemia. Med Oncol 2005;22:217–28.
6. van Dongen JJ, Langerak AW, et al. Design and standardization of PCR primers and protocols for detection of clonal immunoglobulin and T-cell receptor gene recombinations in suspect lymphoproliferations: report of the BIOMED-2 Concerted Action BMH4-CT98-3936. Leukemia 2003;17:2257–317.
7. Bruggemann M, White H, Gaulard P, et al. Powerful strategy for polymerase chain reaction-based clonality assessment in T-cell malignancies. Report of the BIOMED-2 Concerted Action BHM4 CT98-3936. Leukemia 2007;21:215–21.
8. Aster JC, Longtine JA. Detection of BCL2 rearrangements in follicular lymphoma. Am J Pathol 2002;160:759–63.
9. Sherr CJ. Mammalian G1 cyclins. Cell 1993;73:1059–65.
10. Mozos A, Royo C, Hartmann E, et al. SOX11 expression is highly specific for mantle cell lymphoma and identifies the cyclin D1-negative subtype. Haematologica 2009;94:1555–62.
11. Albagli-Curiel O. Ambivalent role of BCL6 in cell survival and transformation. Oncogene 2003;22:507–16.
12. Basso K, Dalla-Favera R. BCL6: master regulator of the germinal center reaction and key oncogene in B cell lymphomagenesis. Adv Immunol 2010;105:193–210.
13. Nakamura N, Nakamine H, Tamaru J, et al. The distinction between Burkitt lymphoma and diffuse large B-Cell lymphoma with c-myc rearrangement. Mod Pathol 2002;15:771–6.
14. Kalla J, Stilgenbauer S, Schaffner C, et al. Heterogeneity of the API2-MALT1 gene rearrangement in MALT-type lymphoma. Leukemia 2000;14:1967–74.
15. Dierlamm J. Genetic abnormalities in marginal zone B-cell lymphoma. Haematologica 2003;88:8–12.

16. Morris SW, Kirstein MN, Valentine MB, et al. Fusion of a kinase gene, ALK, to a nucleolar protein gene, NPM, in non-Hodgkin's lymphoma. Science 1995;267:316–7.
17. Hernandez L, Pinyol M, Hernandez S, et al. TRK-fused gene (TFG) is a new partner of ALK in anaplastic large cell lymphoma producing two structurally different TFG-ALK translocations. Blood 1999;94:3265–8.
18. Breen KA, Grimwade D, Hunt BJ. The pathogenesis and management of the coagulopathy of acute promyelocytic leukaemia. Br J Haematol 2012;156:24–36.
19. De Botton S, Chevret S, Sanz M, et al. Additional chromosomal abnormalities in patients with acute promyelocytic leukaemia (APL) do not confer poor prognosis: results of APL 93 trial. Br J Haematol 2000;111:801–6.
20. Nucifora G, Birn DJ, Erickson P, et al. Detection of DNA rearrangements in the AML1 and ETO loci and of an AML1/ETO fusion mRNA in patients with t(8;21) acute myeloid leukemia. Blood 1993;81:883–8.
21. Le Beau MM, Larson RA, Bitter MA, et al. Association of an inversion of chromosome 16 with abnormal marrow eosinophils in acute myelomonocytic leukemia. A unique cytogenetic-clinicopathological association. N Engl J Med 1983;309:630–6.
22. Kaneko Y, Maseki N, Takasaki N, et al. Clinical and hematologic characteristics in acute leukemia with 11q23 translocations. Blood 1986;67:484–91.
23. Lugthart S, Groschel S, Beverloo HB, et al. Clinical, molecular, and prognostic significance of WHO type inv(3)(q21q26.2)/t(3;3)(q21;q26.2) and various other 3q abnormalities in acute myeloid leukemia. J Clin Oncol 2010;28:3890–8.
24. Grimwade D, Hills RK, Moorman AV, et al. Refinement of cytogenetic classification in acute myeloid leukemia: determination of prognostic significance of rare recurring chromosomal abnormalities among 5876 younger adult patients treated in the United Kingdom Medical Research Council trials. Blood 2010;116:354–65.
25. Marcucci G, Mrozek K, Bloomfield CD. Molecular heterogeneity and prognostic biomarkers in adults with acute myeloid leukemia and normal cytogenetics. Curr Opin Hematol 2005;12:68–75.
26. Faderl S, Talpaz M, Estrov Z, et al. The biology of chronic myeloid leukemia. N Engl J Med 1999;341:164–72.
27. Verfaillie CM. Biology of chronic myelogenous leukemia. Hematol Oncol Clin North Am 1998;12:1–29.
28. Gabert J, Beillard E, van der Velden VH, et al. Standardization and quality control studies of 'real-time' quantitative reverse transcriptase polymerase chain reaction of fusion gene transcripts for residual disease detection in leukemia: a Europe Against Cancer program. Leukemia 2003;17:2318–57.
29. Pozdnyakova O, Miron PM, Tang G, et al. Cytogenetic abnormalities in a series of 1,029 patients with primary myelodysplastic syndromes: a report from the US with a focus on some undefined single chromosomal abnormalities. Cancer 2008;113:3331–40.

Molecular Diagnostics in Colorectal Carcinoma

Amarpreet Bhalla, MBBS, MD[a], Muhammad Zulfiqar, MD[b,*],
Michael Weindel, MD[c], Vinod B. Shidham, MD, FRCPath, FIAC[d]

KEYWORDS

- Chromosomal instability • Microsatellite instability • Methylator phenotype
- CpG island methylator phenotype

KEY POINTS

- Molecular pathogenesis and classification of colorectal carcinoma are based on the traditional adenoma-carcinoma sequence in the Vogelstein model, serrated polyp pathway, and microsatellite instability.
- The genetic basis for hereditary nonpolyposis colorectal cancer is based on detection of mutations in the MLH1, MSH2, MSH6, PMS2. and EPCAM genes.
- Genetic testing for Lynch syndrome includes microsatellite instability testing, methylator phenotype testing, BRAF mutation testing, and molecular testing for germline mutations in MMR genes.
- Molecular makers with predictive and prognostic implications include quantitative multigene reverse transcriptase–polymerase chain reaction assay and KRAS and BRAF mutation analysis.
- Evaluation of potential biomarkers under investigation include one-step nucleic acid amplification and epigenetic inactivation of endothelin 2 and endothelin 3 in colon cancer.
- Molecular screening approaches in colorectal cancer using stool DNA are under investigation.

INTRODUCTION

The pathogenesis of colorectal carcinoma is heterogeneous and involves complex multistep molecular pathways initiated by genetic and epigenetic events. The

[a] Pathology Department, Harper University Hospital, Detroit Medical Center, Wayne State University School of Medicine, 3990 John R Street, Detroit, MI 48201, USA; [b] Cytopathology, Pathology Department, Detroit Medical Center, Wayne State University School of Medicine, Old Hutzel Hospital (Department of Cytology- Ground Floor), 4, 4707 St. Antoine Boulevard, Detroit, MI 48201, USA; [c] Department of Pathology, Karmanos Cancer Center, Detroit Medical Center, Wayne State University School of Medicine, 540 East Canfield, Detroit, MI 48201, USA; [d] Department of Pathology, Karmanos Cancer Center, Detroit Medical Center, Wayne State University School of Medicine, Old Hutzel Hospital (Dept of Cytology- Ground Floor), 4707 St. Antoine Boulevard, Detroit, MI 48201, USA
* Corresponding author.
E-mail address: mzulfiqa@med.wayne.edu

Clin Lab Med 33 (2013) 835–859
http://dx.doi.org/10.1016/j.cll.2013.10.001
labmed.theclinics.com
0272-2712/13/$ – see front matter © 2013 Elsevier Inc. All rights reserved.

attempts to classify the molecular phenotypes of colorectal carcinoma provide the basis for morphologic correlation, categorization of tumor subtypes, and detection of inheritable types. Such studies alert investigators to confounding factors observed in association studies and provide information about potential surrogate markers for clinical and research use. The goal is application of molecular tests for individual patient management. Correlation of pathologic features with various molecular markers will improve clinical outcomes in the near future, especially with evolution of targeted and case-specific therapeutic solutions.[1–3]

EPIDEMIOLOGY

Constitutional (endogenous) as well as environmental (exogenous) factors are associated with the development of colorectal carcinoma. Multiple risk factors and protective factors have been linked to colorectal carcinoma (**Boxes 1** and **2**).

Colorectal carcinoma is more common in late-middle-aged and elderly individuals. Men are at a higher risk for developing this malignancy. There is a strong association with a Western type of diet consisting of high-calorie food, rich in animal fat.[4]

Clinical Features

- Clinical presentation: change in bowel habit, constipation, abdominal distension, hematochezia, tenesmus, weight loss, malaise, fever, anemia.
- Screening: the American Gastroenterological Association, American Medical Association, and American Cancer Society recommend endoscopy with biopsy as the standard screening approach.
- Radiological evaluation by computed tomography scan and magnetic resonance imaging are used to assess locoregional spread and distant metastases.[4–9]

PATHOPHYSIOLOGY AND MOLECULAR GENETICS

The diagrams depict the adenoma-carcinoma sequence and serrated polyp pathway arising from a complex interplay of chromosomal instability, microsatellite instability

---

Box 1
Risk factors for colorectal carcinoma

Family history (first-degree relative)

Physical inactivity (<3 hours per week)

Inflammatory bowel disease (physician-diagnosed Crohn disease, ulcerative colitis, or pancolitis)

Obesity

Red meat/Processed meats

Smoking

Heavy alcohol use

Data from American Cancer Society. Cancer facts & figures 2013. Atlanta (GA): American Cancer Society; 2013. Available at: http://www.cancer.org/cancer/colonandrectumcancer/detailedguide/colorectal-cancer-risk-factors. Accessed May 1, 2013.

(MSI), methylation of CpG islands, KRAS, BRAF, adenomatous polyposis coli (APC), SMAD4, and other point mutations (**Figs. 1–4**).[1]

TRADITIONAL VOGELSTEIN MODEL AND APC GENE PATHWAY

The traditional model of Vogelstein describes the classic adenoma-carcinoma sequence and accounts for approximately 80% of sporadic colon tumors. The pathogenesis involves mutation of the APC gene early in the neoplastic process.[2]

APC Gene

- Tumor suppressor gene
- Location: long (q) arm of chromosome 5 between positions 21 and 22
- Key role in regulating cell division cycle
- Regulates the WNT/β-catenin signaling pathway
- Loss of APC function: β-catenin accumulates and activates the transcription of MYC and cyclin D1 genes, resulting in enhanced proliferation of cells
- Mutations: more than 700 mutations in the APC gene have been identified in familial adenomatous polyposis (FAP), both classic and attenuated types
- FAP: syndrome with inherited truncating APC mutation, leading to the production of an abnormally short, nonfunctional version of the protein, which cannot suppress the cellular overgrowth and leads to the formation of polyps and subsequent progression to carcinoma
- Both copies of the APC gene must be functionally inactivated, either by mutation or by the epigenetic events for development of adenomas; the second allele in adenomas harbors a loss or similar mutation, whereas homozygous deletions of APC are rare or absent
- In sporadic colorectal tumors, the mutation may be in mutation cluster region in APC gene with allelic loss, or mutations may be outside this region with tendency to harbor truncating mutations (**Fig. 5**)[2,3,10]

Neoplastic progression is associated with additional mutations and chromosomal instability, with involvement of:

- KRAS: oncogene: enhances growth and prevent apoptosis
- SMAD2 and SMAD4 (DPC4): tumor suppressor genes: effectors of transforming growth factor β (TGF-β) signaling: allows unrestrained cell growth
- DCC: tumor suppressor gene; location: 18q2.3
- p53: tumor suppressor genes: mutated in 70% to 80% of colon cancers
- Telomerase: increases as lesions become more advanced

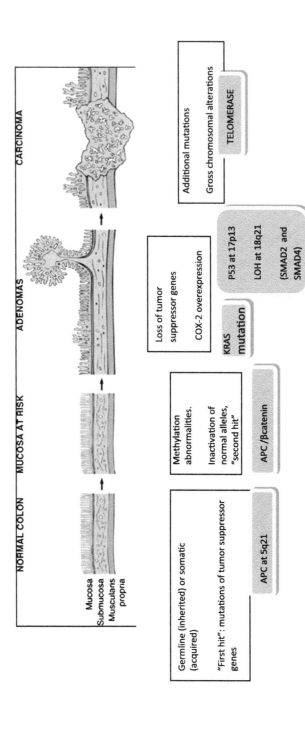

Fig. 1. Adenoma-carcinoma sequence. (*Modified from* Turner JR. The gastrointestinal tract. In: Kumar V, Abbas AK, Fausto N, et al, editors. Robbins and Cotran pathologic basis of disease. 8th edition. Philadelphia: Elsevier; 2010. p. 823; with permission.)

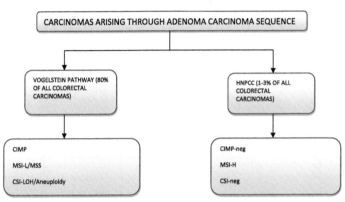

Fig. 2. Subtypes of carcinoma arising through the adenoma-carcinoma sequence.

- Other causes of chromosomal instability: heterogeneous:
Mutations in genes encoding mitosis checkpoint proteins such as BUB1 and BUB1B, abnormal centrosome number, amplification of aurora kinase A (AURKA, STK 15/BTAK), mutations of FBXW7, CHFR.[1,2,11]

Alternatively, tumor suppressor genes may also be silenced by methylation of a CpG-rich zone or CpG island (**Fig. 6**).

HEREDITARY NONPOLYPOSIS COLON CANCER

- The term hereditary nonpolyposis colon cancer (HNPCC) has been used interchangeably with Lynch syndrome.
- Lynch syndrome I is confined to patients presenting only with colorectal cancer (CRC).
- Lynch syndrome II is associated with additional extracolonic cancers.
- HNPCC expresses an autosomal-dominant–like inheritance of colorectal and other cancers with high penetrance.
- It is defined by applying either the Amsterdam I or Amsterdam II criteria and represents about 2% to 3% of all CRCs. An additional 2% to 3% of patients with CRC harbor similar mismatch repair (MMR) gene defects, but do not fulfill the criteria.
- Contrarily, some patients with attenuated FAP-associated and MUTYH-associated polyposis might fulfill Amsterdam criteria for having HNPCC. Revised Bethesda criteria show higher sensitivity in detection of new patients with Lynch syndrome.
- Patients with Lynch syndrome/HNPCC harbor a similar number of adenomatous polyps to the general population. The polyps are indistinguishable from conventional adenomas. Therefore, detection of index cases is challenging and requires the use of specific testing (**Fig. 7**).[5–9,11,12]
- The 4 DNA MMR genes are expressed ubiquitously. They are involved in repair of mismatches resulting from misincorporation, or slippage events, during replication. Hereditary defects in 1 of the 4 MMR genes accounts for 80% to 90% of HNPCC cases.[13–16]
- The MMR gene MSH2 binds with MSH3 and MSH6, forming a functional molecular complex, which facilitates the recognition of the DNA mismatch. Subsequently, the complex recruits MLH1, its binding partner PMS2, and other enzymes, leading to excision, repolymerization, and ligation of the repaired strand of DNA.

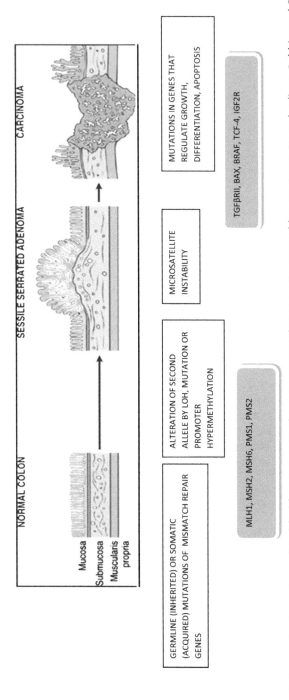

Fig. 3. Serrated polyp pathway. (*Modified from* Turner JR. The gastrointestinal tract. In: Kumar V, Abbas AK, Fausto N, et al, editors. Robbins and Cotran pathologic basis of disease. 8th edition. Philadelphia: Elsevier; 2010. p. 824; with permission.)

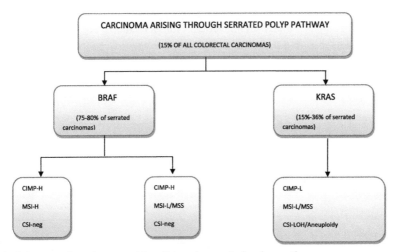

Fig. 4. Subtypes of carcinoma arising through serrated polyp pathway.

- Germline mutations in epithelial cell adhesion molecule (EPCAM) inactivates MSH2 in about 1% of individuals with Lynch syndrome. EPCAM is a calcium-independent cell adhesion membrane protein and is not involved in the physiologic functions of MMR. The EPCAM gene is located on the short (p) arm of chromosome 2 at position 21. Large germline deletions and rearrangement encompassing EPCAM-*MSH2* have been characterized from the 3′ end region of EPCAM to the 5′ initial sequences of the MSH (**Tables 1** and **2**).[12–17]
- The subset of HNPCC cases caused by MMR gene defects is referred to as hereditary MMR deficiency syndrome.
- The MMR-deficient cancers arise after loss of DNA MMR in tumor cells, leading to an increase in the rate of frameshift mutations in microsatellites, designated as MSI.[18,19]
- The frequency of mutations in short repetitive sequences located in coding regions of genes, such as TGFBR2, is also increased.[18–20]
- The germline DNA MMR gene mutations are heterozygous and involve a single allele. The frameshift mutations, nonsense mutations, larger genomic deletions,

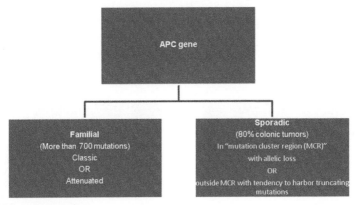

Fig. 5. APC gene mutations.

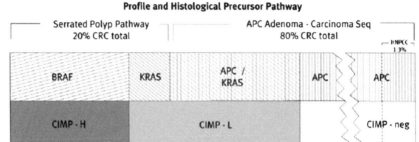

Fig. 6. Molecular genetic profiles of colorectal carcinoma. (*Modified from* O'Brien MJ, Yang S, Huang CS, et al. The serrated polyp pathway to colorectal carcinoma. Mini-symposium: pathology of the large bowel. Diagn Histopathol 2008;14(2):90; with permission.)

and point mutations result in amino acid substitution and premature protein truncation.

- In HNPCC-associated tumors, inactivation of the wild-type allele leads to total loss of DNA MMR activity.
- Genetic instability may operate at the chromosomal level (chromosomal instability), affecting the whole chromosome or parts of chromosomes or at a more

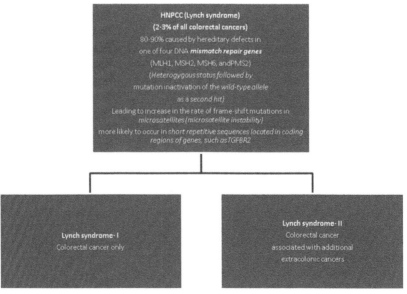

Fig. 7. Lynch syndrome and its types.

Table 1	
Molecular testing for Lynch Syndrome	
Serial Number	**Tests**
1	Evaluation of tumor tissue for MSI: immunohistochemistry for 4 MMR proteins followed by MMR gene mutation testing by PCR
2	Molecular testing of the tumor for methylation abnormalities to rule out sporadic cases
3	Molecular testing of the tumor for BRAF mutations to rule out sporadic cases
4	Molecular genetic testing of the MMR genes to identify germline mutations when findings are consistent with Lynch syndrome

Data from Ref. [4]

subtle level affecting DNA sequences resulting from replication errors (high-frequency MSI [MSI-H]).
- These forms of instability are mutually exclusive, so that CRCs with chromosomal instability are microsatellite stable (MSS) (**Table 3.**).[18–22]
- Appropriate caution must be exercised when correlating single molecular events with patient outcomes. The molecule examined might be associated with global genomic or epigenetic aberrations. and improved or adverse outcomes might be associated with alterations in other molecules.
- Meta-analyses of MSI status and survival of patients with colorectal carcinoma showed that MSI-H tumors were associated with better prognosis compared with MSS tumors.
- MSI-H tumors show no benefit from adjuvant 5-fluorouracil (5-FU).
- Patients with CpG island methylator phenotype (CIMP)-positive tumors experience a significant survival benefit from chemotherapy in contrast to those with CIMP-negative tumors.
- CIMP in non–MSI-H tumors predicts worse survival.[3]

LIMITATIONS OF MOLECULAR CLASSIFICATION AND CORRELATES

- Lack of gold standard and uniform methods, definition, and criteria
- False-positive and false-negative results
- Sampling bias
- Markers used for studies on MSI are not uniform

Table 2	
Genetic basis of HNPCC	
High-Frequency MSI (%)	**Gene Mutation (%)**
Yes (80–90)	*MLH1* (39)
	MSH2 (38)
	MSH6 (11)
	PMS2 (7)
	EPCAM (1)
	Unknown (5)
No (10)	Yes (as above; 10)
	Unknown (90)

Data from Refs. [4,9,15]

Table 3
Molecular pathologic classification of CRC

Group Number	CIMP Status	*MLH1* Status	MSI Status	Chromosomal Status	Precursor	Proportion (%)
1	CIMP high	Full methylation	MSI-H	Stable (diploid)	Serrated polyp	12
2	CIMP high	Partial methylation	MSS/MSI-L Associated with BRAF mutation	Stable (diploid)	Serrated polyp	8
3	CIMP low	No methylation	MSS/MSI-L Associated with KRAS mutation	Unstable (aneuploid)	Adenoma/ serrated polyp	20
4	CIMP negative	No methylation	MSS Associated with KRAS mutation	Unstable (aneuploid)	Adenoma	57
5	CIMP negative	Germline MLH1 or other mutation	MSI-H	Stable (diploid)	Adenoma	3

Abbreviations: CIMP, CpG island methylator phenotype; MSI-L, low-frequency MSI.

Modified from Jass JR. Classification of colorectal cancer based on correlation of clinical, morphological and molecular features. Histopathology 2007;50:119; and *Adapted from* Redston M. Epithelial neoplasms of the large intestine. In: Odze RD, Goldblum JR, editors. Surgical pathology of the GI tract, liver, biliary tract and pancreas. 2nd edition. Elsevier; 2009. p. 597–637.

- Nonuniform methods of detection of methylation markers
- Lack of standardized definition of chromosomal instability[3]

Serrated Polyp Pathway

- The serrated polyp pathway comprises a group of colorectal neoplasms with distinct morphologic and molecular characteristics.
- Aberrant crypt focus (ACF) and hyperplastic polyps comprise the earliest lesions and are associated with activating mutation of the BRAF oncogene. The lesions subsequently progress to sessile serrated adenoma, sessile serrated adenoma with dysplasia, and carcinoma.
- The progress of nondysplastic serrated polyps to more advanced neoplasms is associated with increasing levels of CpG island methylation, leading to inactivation of tumor suppressor genes.
- The carcinomas of this pathway frequently show MSI as a result of epigenetic silencing of hMLH 1.
- **Fig. 8** shows BRAFV600E as an early or instigating mutation originating in a serrated ACF; CpG island methylation is increasing with advancing histologic stage, and MSI-H in later stages, at the interface of serrated adenoma, high-grade dysplasia (HGD) and invasive carcinoma (serrated adenoma/carcinoma [SA/CA]).[1,23]
- Recent studies have shown that transition to HGD and carcinoma is facilitated by methylation-induced silencing of p16 and escape from activation-induced senescence (see **Fig. 8**).[24]
- The other major pathway of pathogenesis of serrated carcinomas arises after KRAS mutations. The carcinomas are microsatellite stable, CIMP low, but show chromosomal instability and loss of heterozygosity of tumor suppressor genes.
- It is one of the earliest genetic mutations in colon carcinogenesis, detected in approximately 40% of the tumors. Along with BRAF mutations, it has been found in the earliest detectable lesions with a serrated morphology. They have been reported in 18% of aberrant crypt foci, 4% to 37% of hyperplastic polyps, 60% of admixed polyps, 80% of traditional serrated adenomas, and up to 10% of sessile serrated adenomas.
- KRAS mutation has been observed to be associated with right-side tumor location. The mutation has significant association with usual tumor histology (vs mucinous, signet ring, medullary), extramural tumor extension, peritumoral

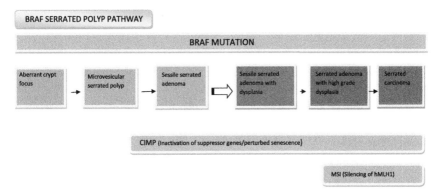

Fig. 8. BRAF serrated polyp pathway. (*Modified from* O'Brien MJ, Yang S, Huang CS, et al. The serrated polyp pathway to colorectal carcinoma. Mini-symposium: pathology of the large bowel. Diagn Histopathol 2008;14(2):79; with permission.)

lymphocytic host response, presence of distant metastases, and absence of lymphovascular invasion at the time of diagnosis.[25–32]

- An unequivocal diagnosis of serrated carcinoma is made when 6 of the 7 histologic criteria listed in **Box 3** are fulfilled.
- The histologic features are similar to those of the conventional adenoma-carcinoma sequence.
- KRAS-mutated traditional serrated adenoma progresses to a mixed tubulovillous adenomatous phenotype and acquires HGD.
- The interface of HGD and infiltrating carcinoma (SA/CA) is associated with p53 mutation.[1,23]
- Traditional serrated adenoma associated with HGD or malignancy is associated with high rates of MLH1 methylation.
- CIMP-H and low tumors are reported with variable frequency (**Fig. 9**)[24]

SPORADIC MSI COLORECTAL CARCINOMA

- MSI is prevalent in 10% to 15% of all colorectal carcinomas.
- Biallelic transcriptional silencing of MLH1 gene secondary to promoter hypermethylation leads to loss of normal MMR function in sporadic colorectal carcinomas. The malignancy develops through the serrated pathway, with sessile serrated adenoma as the precursor lesion.
- The molecular abnormality includes methylation of multiple regions of C-G dinucleotide or CpG islands within the promoter region of genes and subsequent downregulation of these genes. It is known as CIMP and is associated with BRAF mutation in 40% to 50% cases.[33]

PATHOLOGIC FEATURES OF MSI-H COLORECTAL CARCINOMA
Shared by Both Inherited and Sporadic Tumors

- Tendency to occur on right side of colon
- Medullary carcinoma phenotype
- Presence of mucinous or signet ring component
- Presence of tumor infiltrating and peritumoral lymphocytes
- Crohnlike inflammatory response
- Pushing tumor borders (**Fig. 10**)[33]

Box 3
Histomorphologic features of serrated carcinomas

Epithelial serrations

Eosinophilic or clear cytoplasm

Abundant cytoplasm

Vesicular nuclei with peripheral chromatin condensation and a single prominent nucleolus

Distinct nucleoli

Absence of necrosis (or <10% necrosis)

Intracellular and extracellular mucin

Cell balls and papillary rods

Adapted from Bettington M, Walker N, Clouston A, et al. The serrated pathway to colorectal carcinoma: current concepts and challenges. Histopathology 2013;62:382; with permission.

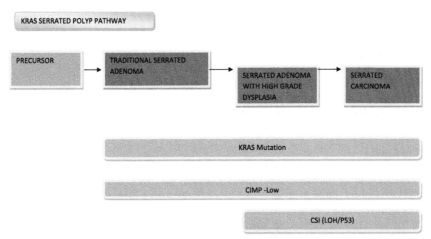

Fig. 9. KRAS serrated polyp pathway. (*Modified from* O'Brien MJ, Yang S, Huang CS, et al. The serrated polyp pathway to colorectal carcinoma. Mini-symposium: pathology of the large bowel. Diagn Histopathol 2008;14(2):79; with permission.)

MMR Testing

Scientific rationale

Patients with HNPCC have tumors with defective DNA MMR and are MSI-H. The MSI-H phenotype can be observed in approximately 15% of sporadic CRC and is not very

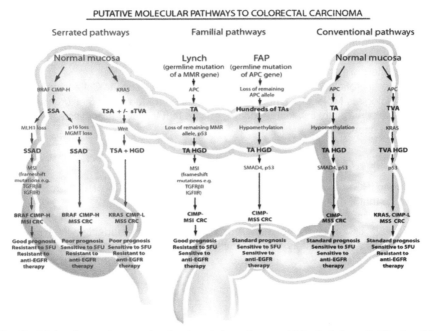

Fig. 10. Molecular pathogenesis of colorectal carcinoma. (*Adapted from* Bettington M, Walker N, Clouston A, et al. The serrated pathway to colorectal carcinoma: current concepts and challenges. Histopathology 2013;62:380; with permission.)

specific for HNPCC. The specificity of MSI testing may be increased by using it primarily on at-risk populations.[34]

Clinical rationale

Germline mutation in one of several DNA MMR genes (eg, MLH1, MSH2, MSH6, or PMS2) may be present in patients with tumors with MSI-H phenotype. Definitive diagnosis of the disorder and presymptomatic detection of carriers in at-risk individuals is possible by follow-up germline testing for HNPCC, with potential reduction in morbidity and mortality.[35]

Best method

MSI testing is generally performed with at least 5 microsatellite markers, generally mononucleotide or dinucleotide repeat markers. In 1998, a National Institutes of Health consensus panel proposed that laboratories use a 5-marker panel comprising 3 dinucleotide and 3 mononucleotide repeats for MSI testing.[36] Because mononucleotide markers have a higher sensitivity and specificity, many commercially available kits use 5 mononucleotide markers.[7,25,35,37–40]

QUALITY ASSURANCE

- The detection of MSI in a tumor by microsatellite analysis requires that the DNA used for the analysis be extracted from a portion of the tumor that contains approximately 40% or more tumor cells.
- Thus, pathologists should help identify areas of the tumor for DNA isolation that have at least this minimum content of tumor cells.
- MSI testing is frequently performed in conjunction with immunohistochemical (IHC) testing for MMR protein expression (ie, MLH1, MSH2, MSH6, and PMS expression).
- If the results of MMR IHC and MSI testing are discordant (eg, MSI-H phenotype with normal IHC or abnormal IHC with MSS phenotype), then the laboratory should make sure that the same sample was used for MSI and IHC testing and that there was no sample mix-up.
- External proficiency testing surveys are available through the College of American Pathologists Molecular Oncology resource committee and other organizations. These surveys are invaluable tools to ensure that the laboratory assays are working as expected.

PITFALLS

- During IHC evaluation of MSI proteins, an intact expression of all 4 proteins indicates that the tested MMR enzymes are intact.
- It is common for intact staining to be patchy.
- Positive IHC reaction for all 4 proteins does not exclude Lynch syndrome, because approximately 5% of families may have a missense mutation (especially in *MLH1*), which can lead to a nonfunctional protein with retained antigenicity.
- Defects in lesser-known MMR enzymes may also lead to a similar result, but this situation is rare.
- Loss of expression of MLH1 may be caused by Lynch syndrome or methylation of the promoter region (as occurs in sporadic MSI colorectal carcinoma). BRAF mutation testing can help in differentiating the cases, although definitive interpretation is possible by genetic testing.[7,25,35,37–40]

Recommendations

- National Comprehensive Cancer Network (NCCN) guidelines recommend MMR protein testing to be performed for all patients younger than 50 years with colon cancer based on an increased likelihood of Lynch syndrome in the US population.
- The testing should also be considered for all patients with stage II disease, because patients with stage II MSI-H may have a good prognosis and do not benefit from 5-FU adjuvant therapy.[19,35,39,40]

MMR IHC

- The DNA MMR proteins are ubiquitously expressed in normal human tissues. HNPCC or Lynch syndrome results in instability of the truncated messenger RNA (mRNA) transcript and the protein product and results in complete loss of ICH-detectable MMR protein in tumors.
- IHC testing is typically performed using antibodies to the 4 genes that harbor the most common known HNPCC mutations: MLH1, MSH2, MSH6, and PMS2.
- Mutation of MLH1 results in its loss from the DNA MMR complex, subsequently leading to loss of PMS2 from the repair protein complex. Therefore, mutation and loss of the MLH1 protein is also usually accompanied by loss of PMS2 expression.
- The same mechanism holds true for MSH2 and its binding partner, MSH6.
- These IHC results are summarized in **Table 4**.
- The specificity of loss of protein expression for an underlying MMR defect is virtually 100%, although up to 10% of these tumors are MSS on MSI testing.
- The staining pattern of the tumor tissue is compared with the normal-appearing control tissue of the same patient to prevent misinterpretation caused by polymorphisms.[4,7,25–29]

MSI TESTING

Frameshift mutations in microsatellites is identified by amplification of selected microsatellites by polymerase chain reaction (PCR) and analysis of fragment size by gel electrophoresis or an automated sequencer after extraction of DNA from both normal and tumor tissue (usually formalin-fixed, paraffin-embedded tissue). The sensitivity of the revised panel of MSI testing is at least 90% (**Table 5**).[4,7,25–28]

Table 4 Interpretation of DNA MMR IHC				
MLH1	**PMS2**	**MSH2**	**MSH6**	**Interpretation**
+	+	+	+	Intact DNA MMR; or rare germline point mutation with intact IHC; or other gene
–	–	+	+	MLH1 methylation silencing or MLH1 germline mutation (HNPCC)
+	+	–	–	MSH2 germline mutation (HNPCC)
+	–	+	+	PMS2 germline mutation (HNPCC) Rare MLH1 mutation may also have this pattern
+	+	+	–	MSH6 germline mutation (HNPCC)

Adapted from Redston M. Epithelial neoplasms of the large intestine. In: Odze RD, Goldblum JR, editors. Surgical pathology of the GI tract, liver, biliary tract and pancreas. 2nd edition. Elsevier; 2009. p. 631; with permission.

Table 5 Bethesda criteria for MSI	
Loci with MSI (%)	Classification
≥40	MSI-H
10–30	MSI-L
0	MSS

Abbreviation: MSI-L, low-frequency MSI.
Adapted from Redston M. Epithelial neoplasms of the large intestine. In: Odze RD, Goldblum JR, editors. Surgical pathology of the GI tract, liver, biliary tract and pancreas. 2nd edition. Elsevier, 2009. p. 629.

Various fluorescent multiplex PCR-based panels (eg, Promega panel) are used for detection of MSI loci. The prototype Promega panel uses fluorescently labeled primers for coamplification of 7 markers for analysis of the MSI-H phenotype, including 5 nearly monomorphic mononucleotide repeat markers (BAT-25, BAT-26, MONO-27, NR-21, and NR-24) and 2 highly polymorphic pentanucleotide repeat markers (Penta C and Penta D). Amplified fragments are detected using special spectral genetic analyzers.[7,26–29]

BRAF Mutation Testing

- BRAF mutations in colorectal carcinoma neoplasms are identical V600E point mutations and are readily assayed by PCR. Mutations in BRAF and KRAS are mutually exclusive and signify resistance to anti–epidermal growth factor receptor (EGFR) antibodies.
- BRAF mutations differentiate sporadic MLH1-deficient (methylated) cancers from hereditary MLH1-deficient cancers with an underlying germline mutation. In MLH1-deficient cancers, *BRAF* mutation testing has a sensitivity of 50% to 70% and a specificity of 100%.
- Use of *BRAF* mutational analysis as a step before germline genetic testing in patients with MSI-H tumors may be a cost-effective means of identifying patients with sporadic tumors, for whom further testing is not indicated.
- BRAF mutations have been reported in 19% to 70% of hyperplastic polyps, in 75% to 82% of sessile serrated adenoma, and in 20% to 66% of traditional serrated adenomas. The presence of BRAF V600E mutation in a microsatellite unstable tumor indicates that the tumor is probably sporadic and not associated with HNPCC.
- In addition, BRAF mutations confer a worse clinical outcome and need for adjuvant therapy. Mutations are associated with reduced overall survival, and shorter progression-free survival. The poor prognosis is attributed to the genetic pathway in which it occurs. The adverse effects are negated in CIMP-positive tumors.[1,25,30–32,41–44]
- There are insufficient data to guide the use of anti-EGFR therapy in the first-line setting with active chemotherapy based on BRAF V600E mutation status.
- The test is performed on formalin-fixed paraffin-embedded tumor tissue by amplification and direct DNA sequence analysis or allele-specific PCR.
- Testing should be performed only in laboratories that are certified under the Clinical Laboratory Improvement Amendments of 1988 (CLIA-88) as qualified to perform high-complexity clinical laboratory (molecular pathology) testing.[1,25,30–32,41–44]

CIMP Testing

- A subset of CRCs (about 25%) have widespread aberrations in DNA methylation, including promoter silencing of genes. Referred to as CIMP, this subset includes most sporadic MSI-H cancers with methylation silencing of MLH1.
- CIMP testing is a method to detect abnormal DNA methylation by using a panel of markers/loci and has been used in some studies to differentiate sporadic from hereditary MLH1-deficient cancers.
- Methylation-specific PCR is widely used for analysis, although there is lack of standardization.
- Although there has not yet been an international consensus on the correct choice of markers for CIMP testing, several loci have begun to emerge as the most sensitive and specific for this type of application.
- Some MSI-H tumors are CIMP-H, but negative for BRAF mutations. Therefore CIMP testing is not a surrogate for BRAF mutation testing and has additional significance.[31,32,41]

KRAS MUTATION TESTING

- Mutations in codons 12 and 13 in exon 2 of the coding region of the KRAS gene predict lack of response to therapy with antibodies targeted to EGFR.
- The presence of the KRAS gene mutation has been shown to be associated with lack of clinical response to therapies targeted at EGFR, such as cetuximab and panitumumab.
- Although clinical guidelines for KRAS mutational analysis are evolving, provisional recommendations from the American Society for Clinical Oncology are that all patients with stage IV colorectal carcinoma who are candidates for anti-EGFR antibody therapy should have their tumor tested for KRAS mutations (http://www.asco.org/, June 2, 2009).
- Testing for mutations in codons 12 and 13 should be performed only in laboratories that are certified under CLIA-88 as qualified to perform high-complexity clinical laboratory (molecular pathology) testing.
- No specific methodology is recommended.
- The testing can be performed on formalin-fixed paraffin-embedded tissue, on primary or metastatic cancer.[23,35,45–47]

REPORTING GUIDELINES (COLLEGE OF AMERICAN PATHOLOGISTS)

- The results of DNA MMR IHC and MSI testing should be incorporated into the surgical pathology report for the CRC case and an interpretation of the clinical significance of these findings provided.
- If DNA MMR IHC has not been performed, this testing should be recommended for any cases that show an MSI-H phenotype, because this information helps identify the gene that is most likely to have a germline mutation.
- Examination of expression of MLH1, MSH2, MSH6, and PMS2 is the most common IHC testing method used for suspected MSI-H cases; antibodies to these MMR proteins are commercially available.
- Any positive reaction in the nuclei of tumor cells is considered as intact expression (normal).
- Loss of MSH2 expression essentially always implies Lynch syndrome.[7,34,35,37–40]

GERMLINE TESTING

HNPCC

- The goal of a genetic workup of families with HNPCC is to identify the underlying germline mutation. Confirmation of the germline mutation allows for the most accurate treatment and follow-up recommendations for the patient, and allows predictive testing to be undertaken in interested family members.
- The initial approach by most laboratories is to analyze the complete coding sequence of the relevant gene or genes (depending on IHC results), as well as a portion of the intronic regions important to exon splicing. Some laboratories use a variety of rapid screening approaches to find mutations, whereas others undertake a complete sequence analysis.[18,28,29]

APC Gene

- Ninety-eight percent of alterations in FAP include frameshift, nonsense, splice site mutations, large deletions, and duplications of the APC gene.
- Testing is performed by mutation screening (Sanger sequencing, conformation sensitive gel electrophoresis, and protein truncation testing) with reflex conformation sequencing.
- Gene deletion or duplication analysis may be performed by multiplex ligation-dependent probe amplification. False-negative results can occur because of deep intronic mutations, allele dropout, somatic mosaicism, and locus heterogeneity for the phenotype.
- Negative results may be followed by MUTYH targeted mutation testing.[26]

ALGORITHMIC STRATEGIES FOR MANAGEMENT OF MMR COLORECTAL CARCINOMA

- There is no definitive standardized practice for triage of colorectal carcinoma for molecular testing. Almost all microsatellite instable colorectal carcinomas are detected by combination of MSI and IHC testing. In the presence of deficient MMR, additional loss of protein expression of MSH2/MSH6, MSH6 alone, or PMS2 increases likelihood of Lynch syndrome.
- Concomitant incidence of defective mismatch repair (dMMR), CIMP-H, and MLH1 supports the diagnosis of sporadic Dmmr CRC.
- Detection of BRAF c.1799T>A mutation serves to exclude diagnosis of Lynch syndrome.
- Funkhauser and colleagues have critically analyzed the various recommendations and have advocated a screening algorithm to include MSI testing, BRAF c. 1799T>A mutation, and IHC for the 4 MMR proteins.
- **Fig. 11** shows MMR subgroup assignment for approximately 94% of colorectal carcinoma cases. Only the MSI-H, MLH1 lost, and BRAF wild-type cases remain unassigned. The group recommends triage of unassigned 6% cases to referral laboratories performing high volumes of hypermethylation, sequencing, and deletion testing for resolution of subgroup assignment.
- An additional subgroup, comprising 1.7% of the cases (those assigned to the Lynch syndrome subgroup), would also be referred to define the germline mutation/deletion involved. The recommendation is based on the expectation that cost of testing is less than cost of delayed diagnosis and absent surveillance of Lynch carriers.[33]
- The NCCN (nccn.org) recommends use of Amsterdam or revised Bethesda criteria as the initial screening step. This approach would miss the diagnosis of

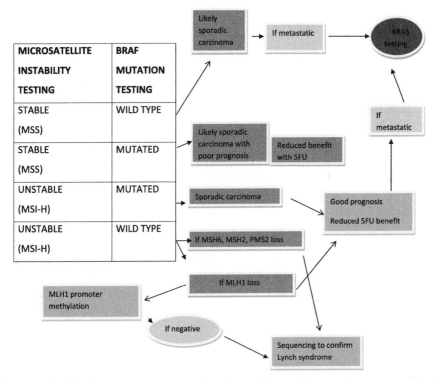

MICROSATELLITE INSTABILITY TESTING	BRAF MUTATION TESTING
STABLE (MSS)	WILD TYPE
STABLE (MSS)	MUTATED
UNSTABLE (MSI-H)	MUTATED
UNSTABLE (MSI-H)	WILD TYPE

Fig. 11. Algorithmic strategies for prognosis and prediction of therapeutic response. (*Modified form* Funkhouser WK Jr, Lubin IM, Monzon FA, et al. Relevance, pathogenesis, and testing algorithm for mismatch repair–defective colorectal carcinomas. A report of the Association for Molecular Pathology. J Mol Diagn 2012;14(2):97, with permission.)

5% to 58% of new Lynch syndrome cases, as well as most sporadic dMMR CRC cases.

- Evaluation of Genomic Applications in Practice and Prevention (EGAPP) estimated detection rates and costs of testing using 4 different testing strategies:
  i. MMR gene sequencing/deletion testing on all probands
  ii. MSI testing, followed by MMR gene sequencing/deletion testing on all MSI-H cases
  iii. IHC testing, with protein loss guiding targeted MMR gene sequencing/deletion testing
  iv. IHC, with BRAF c.1799T>A testing of cases with MLH1 protein loss
  Each of these would fail to detect all dMMR CRC.

- A similar comparison of 4 strategies, each starting with a single test, was recently published by the US Centers for Disease Control and Prevention, with similar limitations to the EGAPP model. The IHC sequencing strategy and IHC_/_ BRAF c.1799T>A sequencing strategy were more cost-effective for diagnosis of Lynch syndrome probands and carriers. However, 11% to 12% of Lynch cases would not be diagnosed because of the absence of MSI testing to identify MSI-H tumors with normal IHC in patients with Lynch syndrome. Published recommendations by other investigators and clinical groups also exist.

- The aim of molecular subgrouping is improved diagnostic accuracy and appropriate therapy, genetic counseling for patients with germline MMR mutations, and appropriate counseling and screening of unaffected family members of patients with Lynch syndrome.[18,33]

MOLECULAR INVESTIGATION OF LYMPH NODES IN PATIENTS WITH COLON CANCER USING ONE-STEP NUCLEIC ACID AMPLIFICATION

A diagnostic system called one-step nucleic acid amplification (OSNA), has recently been designed to detect cytokeratin 19 mRNA as a surrogate for lymph node metastases. In a study by Güller and colleagues,[28] analysis of lymph nodes reported negative after standard hematoxylin-eosin examination resulted in upstaging 2 of 13 patients (15.3%) cases. Compared with histopathology, OSNA had 94.5% sensitivity, 97.6% specificity, and a concordance rate of 97.1%. However, insufficient data are available for routine utilization in standard clinical practice.[48,49]

MOLECULAR STAGING INDIVIDUALIZING CANCER MANAGEMENT

GUCY2C is a member of a family of enzyme receptors synthesizing guanosine $3'5'$cyclic monophosphate from guanosine-$5'$-triphosphate, which is expressed on intestinal epithelial cells but not in extraintestinal tissues. The expression is amplified in colorectal carcinoma compared with normal intestinal tissues. It is identified in all colorectal human tumors independent of anatomic location or grade but not in extragastrointestinal malignancies. Therefore, it has potential application in identifying occult metastases in lymph nodes of patients undergoing staging for CRC. However, there are insufficient data to support its use in standard clinical practice.[50]

NOVEL MOLECULAR SCREENING APPROACHES IN CRC

- Stool DNA (sDNA) potentially offers improved sensitivity, specificity, and cancer prevention by the detection of adenomas. The basis for sDNA screening is the identification of genetic alterations in the initiation of a sequenced progression from adenoma to carcinoma, such as mutations in APC, KRAS, DCC, and p53.
- Key genetic alterations seen in many hereditary forms of CRC correspond to genetic alterations in sporadic CRC, indicating that the somatic occurrence of these genetic alterations leads to the initiation and progression of CRC and supports the targeting of these genes for generalized population screening.
- DNA methylation of CpG islands of known CRC markers has been shown in DNA samples from serum and stool samples of patients with CRC. SFRP2 methylation in fecal DNA was evaluated for detection of hyperplastic and adenomatous colorectal polyps. SFRP methylation was not found in healthy controls.[51]

PREDICTIVE AND PROGNOSTIC MARKERS
Quantitative Multigene Reverse Transcriptase PCR Assay

- Quantitative gene expression assays to assess recurrence risk and benefits from chemotherapy in patients with stage II and III colon cancer have been evaluated and are commercially available. The test provides information on the likelihood of disease recurrence in colon cancer (prognosis) and the likelihood of tumor response to standard chemotherapy regimens (prediction).
- The Oncotype D$_x$ colon cancer assay evaluates a 12-gene panel consisting of 7 cancer genes and 5 reference genes to determine the recurrence score. This score was validated in the QUASAR (Quick and Simple and Reliable) study. The score improves the ability to discriminate high-risk from low-risk patients who have stage II colon cancer beyond known prognostic factors even in the

cohort of apparently low-risk patients. Similar proportional reductions in recurrence risks with 5-FU/leucovorin chemotherapy were observed across the range of recurrence scores.

- Another Oncotype D_x score was validated in the National Surgical Adjuvant Breast and Bowel Project C-07 study, which differentiated risk of recurrence for patients with stage III disease and in the context of oxiplatinin-containing adjuvant therapy[20,29,37,52]

KRAS Mutation

- KRAS mutation has an established role in predicting resistance to anti-EGFR targeted therapy. KRAS gene mutation testing in patients with metastatic colorectal carcinoma guides treatment with anti-EGFR antibody therapy.
- The American Society of Clinical Oncology opines that patients with mutations in codon 12 or 13 (exon 2) should not receive anti-EGFR antibody therapy as part of their treatment. The most commonly used methods to detect the mutations include DNA sequencing (Sanger method or pyrosequencing) and real-time PCR.[53–57]

BRAF Mutation

BRAF is a kinase encoding gene in the RAS/RAF/MAPK pathway. The BRAF V600E mutation signifies resistance to anti-EGFR targeted therapy and may be useful in determining patient eligibility for therapies that target EGFR pathway. The role of BRAF mutations, mutually exclusive with KRAS mutations, in predicting resistance to anti-EGFR monoclonal antibodies is not yet consolidated. There are insufficient data to guide the use of anti-EGFR therapy in the first-line setting with active chemotherapy based on BRAFV600E mutation.[7,35,37,40]

TREATMENT OF COLORECTAL CARCINOMA

- Surgical resection with or without chemotherapy, depending on stage of tumor
- Stage I disease: surgical resection alone
- Stage 4/Duke D, distant metastases: surgery with chemotherapy
- Chemotherapeutic agents used: intravenous 5-FU, oral capecitabine (Xeloda); cytotoxic agents: CPT-11/irinotecan (Campto), a topoisomerase inhibitor, and oxaliplatin (Eloxatin)
- Targeted therapy: humanized anti-EGFR: cetuximab, panitumumab
- Chemotherapeutic and biological compounds are under investigation: tyrosine kinase inhibitors, cyclooxygenase 2 inhibitors, matrix metalloproteinase inhibitors, and various forms of immunotherapy[19,36,39,58–63]

FUTURE TRENDS
Other Gene Mutations Associated with Resistance to Anti-EGFR Therapy[33]

- KRAS mutations at codons 61 and 146
- PIK3CA exon 20 mutation
- PTEN protein inactivation

MicroRNAs
Upregulated microRNAs in colorectal carcinoma miR-96 oncogenic microRNAs (miRNAs) involved in key signaling pathways include miR-96, miR-21, miR-135, and miR17-92 and potentially target CHES1 (transcription factor involved in apoptosis inhibition). miR-21 correlates with the downregulation of tumor suppressor protein

PDCD4. It may target PTEN, a tumor suppressor gene. miR-135a and miR135b correlate with reduced expression of the APC gene. Overexpression of miR17-92 results in suppression of antiangiogenic factors Tsp1 and connective tissue growth factor. It also mediates myc-dependent tumor growth promoting.

Downregulated miRNAs: The downregulated miRNAs include 143 and 145, 31, 96, 133b, 145, and 183. miRNA-133 targets kras, which is known to be involved in signaling pathway for cell proliferation. Expression level of miRNA-31 correlates with development and stage of colorectal carcinoma. Experimentally mediated overexpression of miRNA-34a subsequent effects associated with actions of p53, such as cell cycle arrest and apoptosis, could be phenocopied. There is potential for early detection and staging. It detects precancerous adenomas. It relies on real-time qualitative PCR, which yields results within a 24-hour to 48-hour period.

Limitation It is easily and rapidly degraded by RNases. Determining the oncogenic function of a particular miRNA is difficult, because they target potentially hundreds of oncogenic and antioncogenic gene transcripts.[64]

EPIGENETIC INACTIVATION OF ENDOTHELIN 2 AND ENDOTHELIN 3 IN COLON CANCER

Therapeutic strategies target overexpressed members of the endothelin axis via small molecule inhibitors and receptor antagonists, but this work supports a complementary approach based on the re-expression of endothelin 2 and endothelin 3 as natural antagonists of endothelin 1 in colon cancer.[65]

ACKNOWLEDGMENTS

The authors thank Dr Rish Pai, MD, PhD, Assistant Professor, Department of Pathology, Cleveland Clinic, for his input of this review.

REFERENCES

1. O'Brien MJ, Yang S, Huang CS, et al. The serrated polyp pathway to colorectal carcinoma. Mini-symposium: pathology of the large bowel. Diagn Histopathol 2008;14(2).
2. Vogelstein B, Fearon ER, Stanley SR, et al. Genetic alterations during colorectal tumor development. N Engl J Med 1988;319:525–32.
3. Ogino S, Goel A. Molecular classification and correlates in colorectal cancer. J Mol Diagn 2008;10(1):13–27.
4. Redston M. Epithelial neoplasms of the large intestine. In: Odze RD, Goldblum JR, editors. Surgical pathology of the GI tract, liver, biliary tract and pancreas. 2nd edition. Pennsylvania, Philadelphia: ExpertConsult, Saunders Elsevier; 2004.
5. Omundsen M, Lam FF. The other colonic polyposis syndromes. ANZ J Surg 2012;82:675–81.
6. Lynch HT, Lynch JF. What the physician needs to know about Lynch syndrome: an update. Oncology 2005;19:455–63.
7. Abdel-Rahman WM, Mecklin JP, Peltomaki P. The genetics of HNPCC: application to diagnosis and screening. Crit Rev Oncol Hematol 2006;58:208–20.
8. Gruber SB. New developments in Lynch syndrome (hereditary nonpolyposis colorectal cancer) and mismatch repair gene testing. Gastroenterology 2006; 130:577–87.

9. Woods MO, Williams P, Careen A, et al. A new variant database for mismatch repair genes associated with Lynch syndrome. Hum Mutat 2007; 28:669–73.

10. Rowan AJ, Lamlum H, Ilyas M, et al. APC mutations in sporadic colorectal tumors: a mutational "hotspot" and interdependence of the "two hits". Proc Natl Acad Sci USA 2000;97(7):3352–7.

11. Turner JR. The gastrointestinal tract. In: Kumar V, Abbas AK, Fausto N, et al, editors. Robbins and Cotran pathologic basis of disease. 8th edition. Philadelphia, Pennsylvania: Studentconsult, Suanders Elsevier; 2010. p. 763–832.

12. Umar A, Boland CR, Redston M. Carcinogenesis in the GI tract: from morphology to genetics and back again. Mod Pathol 2001;14:236–45.

13. Pérez-Cabornero L, Infante Sanz M, Velasco Sampedro E, et al. Frequency of rearrangements in Lynch syndrome cases associated with MSH2: characterization of a new deletion involving both EPCAM and the 5' part of MSH2. Cancer Prev Res (Phila) 2011;4:1556–62.

14. Jass JR. Classification of colorectal cancer based on correlation of clinical, morphological and molecular features. Histopathology 2007;50:113–30.

15. Thibodeau SN, Bren G, Schaid D. Microsatellite instability in cancer of the proximal colon. Science 1993;260:816–9.

16. Goel A, Arnold CN, Boland CR. Multistep progression of colorectal cancer in the setting of microsatellite instability: new details and novel insights. Gastroenterology 2001;121:1497–502.

17. Markowitz S, Wang J, Myeroff L, et al. Inactivation of the type II TGF-beta receptor in colon cancer cells with microsatellite instability. Science 1995;268:1336–8.

18. Umar A, Boland CR, Terdiman JP, et al. Revised Bethesda guidelines for hereditary nonpolyposis colorectal cancer (Lynch syndrome) and microsatellite instability. J Natl Cancer Inst 2004;96:261–8.

19. NCCN clinical practice guidelines in oncology (NCCN guidelines). Colon cancer. Version 3. 2013. Available at: nccn.org/professionals/physician_gls/pdf/colon.pdf. Accessed May 2, 2013.

20. Gray R, Barnwell J, McConkey C, et al. Adjuvant chemotherapy versus observation in patients with colorectal cancer: a randomised study. Lancet 2007; 370(9604):2020–9.

21. Bedeir A, Krasinskas AM. Molecular diagnostics of colorectal cancer. Arch Pathol Lab Med 2011;135(5):578–87.

22. Boland CR, Thibodeau SN, Hamilton SR, et al. A National Cancer Institute Workshop on Microsatellite Instability for cancer detection and familial predisposition: development of international criteria for the determination of microsatellite instability in colorectal cancer. Cancer Res 1998;58:5248–57.

23. O'Brien MJ. Hyperplastic and serrated polyps of the colorectum. Gastroenterol Clin North Am 2007;36:947–68.

24. Bettington M, Walker N, Clouston A, et al. The serrated pathway to colorectal carcinoma: current concepts and challenges. Histopathology 2013;62:367–86.

25. Rajagopalan H, Bardelli A, Lengauer C, et al. Tumorigenesis: RAF/RAS oncogenes and mismatch-repair status. Nature 2002;418:934.

26. Kerr SE, Thomas CB, Thibodeau SN, et al. APC germline mutations in individuals being evaluated for familial adenomatous polyposis. A review of the Mayo Clinic experience with 1591 consecutive tests. J Mol Diagn 2013;15(1):31–43.

27. Smyrk TC, Watson P, Kaul K, et al. Tumor-infiltrating lymphocytes are a marker for microsatellite instability in colorectal carcinoma. Cancer 2001;91: 2417–22.

28. Güller U, Zettl A, Worni M, et al. Molecular investigation of lymph nodes in colon cancer patients using one-step nucleic acid amplification (OSNA). Cancer 2012;118:6039–45.

29. Kuebler JP, Wieand HS, O'Connell MJ, et al. Oxaliplatin combined with weekly bolus fluorouracil and leucovorin as surgical adjuvant chemotherapy for stage II and III colon cancer: results from NSABP C-07. J Clin Oncol 2007;25(16):2198–204.

30. Davies H, Bignell GR, Cox C, et al. Mutations of the BRAF gene in human cancer. Nature 2002;417:949–54.

31. Toyota M, Ahuja N, Ohe-Toyota M, et al. CpG island methylator phenotype in colorectal cancer. Proc Natl Acad Sci U S A 1999;96:8681–6.

32. Weisenberger DJ, Siegmund KD, Campan M, et al. CpG island methylator phenotype underlies sporadic microsatellite instability and is tightly associated with BRAF mutation in colorectal cancer. Nat Genet 2006;38:787–93.

33. Funkhouser WK Jr, Lubin IM, Monzon FA, et al. Relevance, pathogenesis, and testing algorithm for mismatch repair-defective colorectal carcinomas. A report of the Association for Molecular Pathology. J Mol Diagn 2012;14(2):91–103.

34. Marcus VA, Madlensky L, Gryfe R, et al. Immunohistochemistry for hMLH1 and hMSH2: a practical test for DNA mismatch repair-deficient tumors. Am J Surg Pathol 1999;23:1248–55.

35. Ribic CM, Sargent DJ, Moore MJ, et al. Tumor microsatellite-instability status as a predictor of benefit from fluorouracil-based adjuvant chemotherapy for colon cancer. N Engl J Med 2003;249(3):247–57.

36. Popovici V, Budinska E, Tejpar S, et al. Identification of a poor-prognosis BRAF-mutant–like population of patients with colon cancer. J Clin Oncol 2012;20: 1288–95.

37. QUASAR: a randomized study of adjuvant chemotherapy (CT) vs observation including 3238 colorectal cancer patients. Journal of Clinical Oncology, 2004 ASCO Annual Meeting Proceedings (Post-Meeting Edition) 2004;22(14S (July 15 Supplement)):3501.

38. Sargent DJ, Marsoni S, Monges G, et al. Defective mismatch repair as a predictive marker for lack of efficacy of fluorouracil-based adjuvant therapy in colon cancer. J Clin Oncol 2010;28(20):3219–26.

39. Stack E, Dubois RN. Role of cyclooxygenase inhibitors for the prevention of colorectal cancer. Gastroenterol Clin North Am 2001;30:1001–10.

40. Thibodeau SN, French AJ, Roche PC, et al. Altered expression of hMSH2 and hMLH1 in tumors with microsatellite instability and genetic alterations in mismatch repair genes. Cancer Res 1996;56:4836–40.

41. Shen L, Toyota M, Kondo Y, et al. Integrated genetic and epigenetic analysis identifies three different subclasses of colon cancer. Proc Natl Acad Sci U S A 2007;104:18654–9.

42. Stefanius K, Ylitalo L, Tuomisto A, et al. Frequent mutations of KRAS in addition to BRAF in colorectal serrated adenocarcinoma. Histopathology 2011;58:679–92.

43. Loupakis F, Ruzzo A, Cremolini C, et al. KRAS codon 61, 146 and BRAF mutations predict resistance to cetuximab plus irinotecan in kras codon 12 and 13 wild-type metastatic colon cancer. Br J Cancer 2009;101:715–21.

44. Spring KJ, Zhao ZZ, Karamatic RR. High prevalence of sessile serrated adenomas with BRAF mutations: a prospective study of patients undergoing colonoscopy. Gastroenterology 2006;131(5):1400–7.

45. Amado RG, Wolf M, Peeters M, et al. Wild-type KRAS is required for panitumumab efficacy in patients with metastatic colorectal cancer. J Clin Oncol 2008;26: 1626–34.

46. Lievre A, Bachet JB, Boige V, et al. KRAS mutations as an independent prognostic factor in patients with advanced colorectal cancer treated with cetuximab. J Clin Oncol 2008;26:374–9.
47. Wijesuriya RE, Deen KI, Hewavisenthi J, et al. Neoadjuvant therapy for rectal cancer down-stages the tumor but reduces lymph node harvest significantly. Surg Today 2005;35(6):442–5.
48. Lindor NM, Burgart LJ, Leontovich O, et al. Immunohistochemistry versus microsatellite instability testing in phenotyping colorectal tumors. J Clin Oncol 2002; 20:1043–8.
49. Lagerstedt Robinson K, Liu T, Vandrovcova J, et al. Lynch syndrome (hereditary nonpolyposis colorectal cancer) diagnostics. J Natl Cancer Inst 2007;99:291–9.
50. Mejia A, Schulz S, Hyslop T, et al. Molecular staging individualizing cancer management. J Surg Oncol 2012;105:468–74.
51. Miller S, Steele S. Novel molecular screening approaches in colorectal cancer. J Surg Oncol 2012;105:459–67.
52. O'Connell MJ, Laurie JA, Kahn M, et al. Prospectively randomized trial of postoperative adjuvant chemotherapy in patients with high risk colon cancer. J Clin Oncol 1998;16:295–300.
53. Gunal A, Hui P, Kilic S, et al. KRAS mutations are associated with specific morphologic features in colon cancer. J Clin Gastroenterol 2013;47(6):509–14.
54. Javle M, Hsueh CT. Updates in gastrointestinal oncology–insights from the 2008 44th annual meeting of the American Society of Clinical Oncology. J Hematol Oncol 2009;2:9.
55. Rizzo S, Bronte G, Fanale D, et al. Prognostic vs predictive molecular biomarkers in colorectal cancer: is KRAS and BRAF wild type status required for anti-EGFR therapy? Cancer Treat Rev 2010;36(Suppl 3):S56–61. http://dx.doi.org/10.1016/S0305-7372(10)70021-9.
56. Andreyev HJ, Norman AR, Cunningham D, et al. Kirsten ras mutations in patients with colorectal cancer: the "RASCAL II" study. Br J Cancer 2001;85:692–6.
57. Keller JW, Franklin JL, Graves-Deal R, et al. Oncogenic KRAS provides a uniquely powerful and variable oncogenic contribution among RAS family members in the colonic epithelium. J Cell Physiol 2007;210:740–9.
58. American Cancer Society. Cancer facts & figures 2013. Atlanta (GA): American Cancer Society; 2013. Available at: http://www.cancer.org/cancer/colonandrectumcancer/detailedguide/colorectal-cancer-risk-factors.
59. Di Nicolantonio F, Martini M, Molinari F, et al. Wild-type BRAF is required for response to panitumumab or cetuximab in metastatic colorectal cancer. J Clin Oncol 2008;26:5705–12.
60. Chan TA. Nonsteroidal anti-inflammatory drugs, apoptosis, and colon-cancer chemoprevention. Lancet Oncol 2002;3:166–74.
61. Gwyn K, Sinicrope FA. Chemoprevention of colorectal cancer. Am J Gastroenterol 2002;97:13–21.
62. Tebbutt NC, Cattell E, Midgley R, et al. Systemic treatment of colorectal cancer. Eur J Cancer 2002;38:1000–15.
63. Wolpin BM, Meyerhardt JA, Mamon HJ, et al. Adjuvant treatment of colorectal cancer. CA Cancer J Clin 2007;57:168–85.
64. Menéndez P, Villarejo P, Padilla D, et al. Diagnostic and prognostic significance of serum MicroRNAs in colorectal cancer. J Surg Oncol 2013;107:217–20.
65. Wang R, Löhr CV, Fischer K, et al. Epigenetic inactivation of endothelin-2 and endothelin-3 in colon cancer. Int J Cancer 2012;132:1004–12.

Molecular Diagnostics in the Neoplasms of Small Intestine and Appendix

Amarpreet Bhalla, MBBS, MD[a], Muhammad Zulfiqar, MD[b],*,
Michael Weindel, MD[c], Vinod B. Shidham, MD, FRCPath, FIAC[d]

KEYWORDS

- Microsatellite instability • KRAS • BRAF • Small intestine • Appendix

KEY POINTS

- Adenocarcinoma of the small intestine arises through adenoma-carcinoma sequence as described by Vogelstein in the colon.
- Adenocarcinomas arising in the background of inflammatory bowel disease develop through the dysplasia-carcinoma sequence.
- β-Catenin mutation is reported in 54% cases.
- Microsatellite instability has been reported in 18% to 35% of small bowel adenocarcinomas.
- Molecular makers with predictive and prognostic implications include quantitative multi-gene reverse transcriptase-polymerase chain reaction assay and KRAS and BRAF mutation analysis.

INTRODUCTION

Adenocarcinoma of the small intestine is relatively rare in comparison to colorectal carcinoma. Some clinical conditions are associated with adenocarcinoma and are listed in **Box 1**. Adenocarcinoma of the small intestine arises through the adenoma-carcinoma sequence as described by Vogelstein in the colon. However, adenocarcinomas arising in the background of inflammatory bowel disease develop through the dysplasia-carcinoma sequence.[1,2] Most of the cases occur in the duodenum;

[a] Department of Pathology, PGY-3 Detroit Medical Center, Harper University Hospital, Wayne State University School of Medicine, 3990 John R Street, Detroit, MI 48201, USA; [b] Department of Pathology and Laboratory Medicine, Indiana University School of Medicine, 350 West 11th Street, Indianapolis, IN 46202-3082, USA; [c] Department of Pathology, Karmanos Cancer Center, Detroit Medical Center, Wayne State University School of Medicine, 540 East Canfield, Detroit, MI 48201, USA; [d] Department of Pathology, Karmanos Cancer Center, Detroit Medical Center, Wayne State University School of Medicine, Old Hutzel Hospital (Dept of Cytology- Ground Floor), 4707 Saint Antoine Boulevard, Detroit, MI 48201, USA
* Corresponding author.
E-mail addresses: mzulfiqa@iupui.edu; mizulfiqar@gmail.com

Clin Lab Med 33 (2013) 861–866
http://dx.doi.org/10.1016/j.cll.2013.08.007
0272-2712/13/$ – see front matter © 2013 Elsevier Inc. All rights reserved.

Box 1
Conditions associated with increased risk of small intestine adenocarcinoma

Sporadic adenomatous polyps

Congenital anomalies

Long-standing ileostomy

Crohn disease

Celiac disease

α-Chain disease

Familial adenomatous polyposis

Gardner syndrome

Peutz-Jeghers syndrome

Hereditary nonpolyposis colon cancer syndrome (Lynch syndrome)

Juvenile polyposis syndrome

Adapted from Noffsinger A. Chapter 22: epithelial neoplasms of the small intestine. In: Odze RD, Goldblum JR, editors. Surgical pathology of the GI tract, liver, biliary tract and pancreas. 2nd edition. Elsevier; 2009. Expertconsult. Copyright © 2009, 2004 by Saunders, an imprint of Elsevier Inc; with permission.

---

however, adenocarcinoma occurring in association with Crohn disease is more common in the ileum.[2]

EPIDEMIOLOGY

- Small intestinal adenocarcinomas usually present between 60 and 70 years of age. Patients with hereditary cancer syndromes present at a younger age.
- The age-adjusted incidence rate of appendiceal adenocarcinoma is 0.2 per 100,000 per annum in the Surveillance, Epidemiology, and End Results study in North America. A slight male predominance has been reported. The median age at presentation is 65 years.[3–5]

SMALL INTESTINAL ADENOCARCINOMA ASSOCIATED WITH CELIAC DISEASE

Small intestinal adenocarcinoma has been reported to arise in the small intestine of celiac disease patients and follows the adenoma-carcinoma sequence.[6,7]

APPENDICEAL ADENOCARCINOMA

Malignant epithelial tumors of the appendix include low-grade appendiceal mucinous neoplasm, adenocarcinoma and carcinoid tumor.[2]

AMPULLARY ADENOCARCINOMA

Most ampullary adenocarcinomas are the intestinal type. The remainder are pancreatobiliary type. Mucinous, signet ring, clear cell, and neuroendocrine have also been reported.[5,8–11]

Ampullary adenocarcinomas have a better prognosis than distal tumors because they become symptomatic early and must be removed at a less advanced stage of growth.[2,12–14]

MUTATIONS

1. Tp53 is a late event in the adenoma-carcinoma sequence and is identified in 20% to 53% of cases.[15]
2. Kirsten rat sarcoma viral oncogene homolog (v-Ki-ras2 or KRAS) transmits signals from extracellular growth factors to cell nucleus. Mutations in this protein are found in colorectal adenomas and adenocarcinomas. Mutations have also been reported in 14% to 83% cases of small intestinal adenocarcinoma, suggesting an adenoma-carcinoma sequence similar colon cancer.[15–18]
3. APC and β-catenin are important proteins in the Wnt pathway. APC mutations are rare in small intestinal adenocarcinoma. The β-catenin mutation is relatively commonly reported in 54% of small intestinal adenocarcinomas.[19]
4. Mismatch repair (MMR) genes: Small bowel adenocarcinomas are known to occur with increased frequency in patients with hereditary nonpolyposis colorectal cancer (HNPCC). Microsatellite instability (MSI) has been reported in 18% to 35% of small bowel adenocarcinomas.[20–24]
5. The tumor suppressor protein Smad4 (mothers against decapentaplegic; Darfwin family of proteins that modulate members of the TGFβ protein superfamily [deleted in pancreatic cancer, locus 4, DPC4]) has been reported in 24% of small intestinal nonampullary adenocarcinomas.[25]
6. Vascular endothelial growth factor A (VEGF-A) and epidermal growth factor receptor (EGFR) may be identified in up to 71% cases, suggesting a potential benefit from anti-EGFR therapy.[24]

MUTATIONS IN APPENDICEAL CARCINOMA

1. Appendiceal carcinomas display serrated architecture but have a low frequency of MSI.
2. Kras mutation is frequent.
3. Loss of 18q is common.
4. Mutation of DPC4 might be associated.
5. In comparison to colonic adenocarcinomas, the tumors have a lower proliferation fraction, apoptotic count, and CD44 expression.[4]

Management Guidelines

- In the case of incidentally discovered epithelial appendiceal neoplasms, colonoscopy is performed to exclude the possibility of synchronus lesions.
- The National Comprehensive Cancer Network management guidelines recommend treatment of small intestinal and appendiceal adenocarcinomas with systemic chemotherapy in accordance with National Comprehensive Cancer Network guidelines for colon cancer.[23] Testing for MSI, KRAS, and v-Raf murine sarcoma viral oncogene homolog B1 (BRAF)V600E mutations may be carried out on formalin-fixed paraffin embedded tumor tissue accordingly.

MOLECULAR TESTING
MSI

Mismatch repair (MMR) protein expression testing by immunohistochemistry for MLH1, PMS2, MSH6, and MSH2 may be followed by microsatellite instability testing of mutations by PCR.[24]

Screening patients with small intestine cancer
Patients at risk for HNPCC can be tested for MSI cost-effectively. MSI-H phenotype implies possible germline mutation in one of several DNA MMR genes (eg, *MLH1*, *MSH2*, *MSH6*, or *PMS2*). Screening for the germline mutation may be considered after appropriate genetic counseling.

Follow-up germline testing for HNPCC
Follow up germline testing for HNPCC helps in making a definitive diagnosis of the disorder and aids in the early detection of carriers, thereby reducing the morbidity, mortality and health care costs.

Pitfalls

1. During immunohistochemical evaluation of MSI proteins, an intact expression of all 4 proteins indicates that MMR enzymes tested are intact but does not entirely exclude Lynch syndrome, because approximately 5% of families may have a missense mutation (especially in *MLH1*) that can lead to a nonfunctional protein with retained antigenicity.
2. Defects in lesser known MMR enzymes may also lead to a similar result, but this situation is rare.
3. Loss of expression of MLH1 may be due to Lynch syndrome or methylation of the promoter region (as occurs in sporadic MSI colorectal carcinoma).
4. BRAF mutation testing can help in differentiating the cases, although definitive interpretation is possible by genetic testing.
5. Loss of MSH2 expression usually implies Lynch syndrome.
6. PMS2 loss is often associated with loss of MLH1 and is only independently meaningful if MLH1 is intact. MSH6 is similarly related to MSH2.[21,26,27]

KRAS

Mutations in codons 12 and 13 in exon 2 of the coding region of KRAS gene predict a lack of response to therapy with antibodies targeted to EGFR. Testing for mutations in codons 12 and 13 should be performed only in laboratories that are certified under the clinical laboratory improvement amendments of 1988 (CLIA-88) as qualified to perform high-complexity clinical laboratory (molecular pathology) testing. No specific methodology is recommended.

The testing can be performed on formalin-fixed paraffin embedded tissue, on primary or metastatic cancer.[21,23,26–28]

BRAF

Patients with BRAFV600E mutations have a poor prognosis. There are insufficient data to guide the use of anti-EGFR therapy in the first-line setting with active chemotherapy based on BRAFV600E mutation status. The test is performed on formalin-fixed paraffin embedded tumor tissue by amplification and direct DNA sequence analysis or allele-specific PCR. Testing should be performed only in laboratories that are certified under the clinical laboratory improvement amendments of 1988 (CLIA-88) as qualified to perform high-complexity clinical laboratory (molecular pathology) testing.[8,9,28–31]

Quality assurance (College of American Pathologists [CAP] guidelines)

- The detection of MSI in a tumor by microsatellite analysis requires that the DNA used for the analysis be extracted from a portion of the tumor that contains approximately $\geq$40% tumor cells. Thus, pathologists should help identify areas of the tumor for DNA isolation that have at least this minimum content of tumor cells.

- MSI testing is frequently performed in conjunction with immunohistochemical (IHC) testing for MMR protein expression (ie, MLH1, MSH2, MSH6, and PMS expression).
- If the results of MMR IHC and MSI testing are discordant (eg, MSI-H phenotype with normal IHC or abnormal IHC with MSS phenotype), then the laboratory should make sure that the same sample was used for MSI and IHC testing and that there was no sample mix-up.
- College of American Pathologists proficiency testing is available through the CAP Molecular Oncology Resource committee.[21,26,27]

REFERENCES

1. Vogelstein B, Fearon ER, Stanley SR, et al. Genetic alterations during colorectal tumor development. N Engl J Med 1988;319:525–32.
2. Noffsinger A. Epithelial neoplasms of the small intestine. In: Odze RD, Goldblum JR, editors. Surgical pathology of the GI tract, liver, biliary tract and pancreas. Philadelphia, PA: Saunders Elsevier; 2009. p. 581–96.
3. Thomas RM, Sobin LH. Gastrointestinal cancer: incidence and prognosis by histologic type: SEER population-based data, 1973–1987. Cancer 1995;75(1): 154–70.
4. Misdraji J, Burgart LJ, Lauwers GY. Defective mismatch repair in the pathogenesis of low-grade appendiceal mucinous neoplasms and adenocarcinomas. Mod Pathol 2004;17:1447–54.
5. Maru D, Wu TT, Canada A, et al. Loss of chromosome 18q and DPC4 (Smad4) mutations in appendiceal adenocarcinomas. Oncogene 2004;23:859–64.
6. Straker RJ, Gunasekaran S, Brady PG. Adenocarcinoma of the jejunum in association with celiac sprue. J Clin Gastroenterol 1989;11:320–3.
7. Rampertab SD, Forde KA, Green PH. Small bowel neoplasia in coeliac disease. Case report. Gut 2003;52:1211–4.
8. Popovici V, Budinska E, Tejpar S, et al. Identification of a poor-prognosis BRAF-mutant–like population of patients with colon cancer. J Clin Oncol 2012;30: 1288–95.
9. Di Nicolantonio F, Martini M, Molinari F, et al. Wild-type BRAF is required for response to panitumumab or cetuximab in metastatic colorectal cancer. J Clin Oncol 2008;26:5705–12.
10. Mitomi H, Nakamura T, Ihara A, et al. Frequent Ki-ras mutations and transforming growth factor-α expression in adenocarcinomas of the small intestine: report of 7 cases. Dig Dis Sci 2003;48:203–9.
11. Lynch HT, Smyrk TC, Lynch PM, et al. Adenocarcinoma of the small bowel in Lynch syndrome II. Cancer 1989;64:2178–83.
12. Baczako K, Buchler M, Beger HG, et al. Morphogenesis and possible precursor lesions of invasive carcinoma of the papilla of Vater: epithelial dysplasia and adenoma. Hum Pathol 1985;16:305–10.
13. Kimura W, Futakawa N, Yamagata S, et al. Different clinicopathologic findings in two histologic types of carcinoma of papilla of Vater. Jpn J Cancer Res 1994;85:161–5.
14. Talbot IC, Neoptolemos JP, Shaw DE, et al. The histopathology and staging of carcinoma of the ampulla of Vater. Histopathology 1988;12:155–65.
15. Arai M, Shimizu S, Imai Y, et al. Mutations of the Ki-ras, p53 and APC genes in adenocarcinomas of the human small intestine. Int J Cancer 1997;70:390–5.

16. Arber N, Shapira I, Ratan J, et al. Activation of c-kras mutations in human gastro-intestinal tumors. Gastroenterology 2000;118:1045–50.

17. Sutter T, Arber N, Moss SF, et al. Frequent K-ras mutations in small bowel adeno-carcinomas. Dig Dis Sci 1996;41:115–8.

18. Younes N, Fulton N, Tanaka R, et al. The presence of K-12 ras mutations in duodenal adenocarcinomas and the absence of ras mutations in other small bowel adenocarcinomas and carcinoid tumors. Cancer 1997;79:1804–8.

19. Wheeler JM, Warren BF, Mortensen NJ, et al. An insight into the genetic pathway of adenocarcinoma of the small intestine. Gut 2002;50:218–23.

20. Benatti P, Roncucci L, Percesepe A, et al. Small bowel carcinoma in hereditary nonpolyposis colorectal cancer. Am J Gastroenterol 1998;93:2219–22.

21. Planck M, Ericson K, Piotrowska Z, et al. Microsatellite instability and expression of MLH1 and MSH2 in carcinomas of the small intestine. Cancer 2003;97:1551–7.

22. Vasen HF, Wijnen JT, Menko FH, et al. Cancer risk in families with hereditary non-polyposis colorectal cancer diagnosed by mutation analysis. Gastroenterology 1996;110:1020–7.

23. Rashid A, Hamilton SR. Genetic alterations in sporadic and Crohn's associated adenocarcinomas of the small intestine. Gastroenterology 1997;113:127–35.

24. Overman MJ, Pozadzides J, Kopetz1 S, et al. Immunophenotype and molecular characterisation of adenocarcinoma of the small intestine. Br J Cancer 2010;102:144–50.

25. Blaker H, von Herbay A, Penzel R, et al. Genetics of adenocarcinomas of the small intestine: frequent deletions at chromosome 18q and mutations of the SMAD4 gene. Oncogene 2002;21:158.

26. Brueckl WM, Heinze E, Milsmann C, et al. Prognostic significance of microsatellite instability in curatively resected adenocarcinoma of the small intestine. Cancer Lett 2004;203:181–90.

27. Boland CR, Thibodeau SN, Hamilton SR, et al. A National Cancer Institute Work-shop on Microsatellite Instability for cancer detection and familial predisposition: development of international criteria for the determination of microsatellite instability in colorectal cancer. Cancer Res 1998;58:5248–57.

28. Amado RG, Wolf M, Peeters M, et al. Wild-type KRAS is required for panitumumab efficacy in patients with metastatic colorectal cancer. J Clin Oncol 2008;26:1626–34.

29. NCCN Clinical Practice Guidelines in Oncology. (NCCN Guidelines). Colon cancer. Version 3. 2013. Available at: nccn.org. Accessed September 7, 2013.

30. Sargent DJ, Marsoni S, Monges G. Defective mismatch repair as a predictive marker for lack of efficacy of fluorouracil-based adjuvant therapy in colon cancer. J Clin Oncol 2010;28(20):3219–26.

31. Lievre A, Bachet JB, Boige V, et al. KRAS mutations as an independent prog-nostic factor in patients with advanced colorectal cancer treated with cetuximab. J Clin Oncol 2008;26:374–9.

Molecular Diagnostics in Esophageal and Gastric Neoplasms

Muhammad Zulfiqar, MD[a],*, Amarpreet Bhalla, MBBS, MD[b],
Michael Weindel, MD[c], Vinod B. Shidham, MD, FRCPath, FIAC[d]

KEYWORDS

- Esophagus • Squamous cell carcinoma • Adenocarcinoma • Gastric carcinoma
- Molecular genetics • HER-2 • Trastuzumab

KEY POINTS

- Esophageal carcinoma (EC) is rapidly increasing in incidence in the United States.
- Barrett esophagus is an established precursor lesion for esophageal adenocarcinoma.
- Genetic changes associated with the development of EC involve the p16, p53, and APC genes.
- Human epidermal growth factor 2 (HER-2) overexpression is seen in gastroesophageal junction carcinoma and a subset gastric carcinoma (GC).
- Trastuzumab is the first FDA-approved target agent for treatment of patients with HER-2 amplified cancers.
- HER-2 overexpression can be detected using immunohistochemistry, fluorescence in situ hybridization, or silver in situ hybridization.
- Other genetic changes seen in GC include chromosome gains and losses, microsatellite instability, changes in expression of vascular endothelial growth factor expression, cyclin E, retinoblastoma, p53, and Protection of telomeres 1.

INTRODUCTION

Esophageal carcinoma (EC) is the most rapidly increasing tumor in incidence in the United States. It has an established association with a precursor lesion (Barrett esophagus). Gastric carcinoma (GC) is the second leading cause of cancer death in the

[a] Department of Pathology and Laboratory Medicine, Indiana University School of Medicine, 350 West 11th Street, Indianapolis, IN 46202-3082, USA; [b] Pathology Department, Harper University Hospital, PGY-3 Detroit Medical Center, Wayne State University School of Medicine, 3990 John R Street, Detroit, MI 48201, USA; [c] Department of Pathology, Karmanos Cancer Center, Detroit Medical Center, Wayne State University School of Medicine, 540 East Canfield, Detroit, MI 48201, USA; [d] Department of Pathology, Karmanos Cancer Center, Detroit Medical Center, Wayne State University School of Medicine, Old Hutzel Hospital (Department of Cytology-Ground Floor), 4707 Street Antoine Boulevard, Detroit, MI 48201, USA
* Corresponding author.
E-mail addresses: mzulfiqa@iupui.edu; mizulfiqar@gmail.com

Clin Lab Med 33 (2013) 867–873
http://dx.doi.org/10.1016/j.cll.2013.08.006
labmed.theclinics.com
0272-2712/13/$ – see front matter © 2013 Elsevier Inc. All rights reserved.

world. Up to half of the cases of GC are related to *Helicobacter pylori* infection.[1–5] The prognosis for patients with advanced stage GC and EC is poor. Human epidermal growth factor 2 (HER-2) overexpression is seen in gastroesophageal junction (GEJ) carcinoma and a subset of GC. HER-2 overexpressing tumors are eligible for HER-2-targeted therapies, which leads to a better survival in these patients.

EPIDEMIOLOGY

EC is the sixth leading cause of cancer death worldwide.[6] The tumors evolve through a pathway from metaplasia (Barrett esophagus) to dysplasia and finally to cancer.[7]

Two subtypes of EC, squamous cell carcinoma and adenocarcinoma (ADC), differ in the incidence and distribution of disease.[6] Squamous cell EC is more prevalent in the Asia Pacific region, whereas ADC is more common in the western world. Esophageal cancer is common in men more than 50 years of age with a strong Caucasian prevalence.

Squamous cell EC is related to smoking and alcohol, whereas Barrett esophagus, caused by gastroesophageal reflux disease (GERD), is the risk factor for ADC.[7]

The incidence of GC is the highest in Eastern Asia, Eastern Europe, and South America.[8] Distal stomach tumors are more common in Asia and tend to have a favorable outcome with surgery,[9] compared with gastric cardia tumors, which are more common in US patients.[8]

Diffuse GC has a hereditary form and results from E-cadherin (CDH1) deregulation, whereas occurrence of intestinal type is associated with environmental factors, such as obesity, dietary factors, cigarette smoking, as well as with infection by *H pylori*.

CLINICAL FEATURES

EC presents with obstructive symptoms including dysphagia and odynophagia. Weight loss is also common. Most patients with GC are asymptomatic. Epigastric pain and dyspepsia are the most frequent symptoms. Most tumors are located on the lesser curvature and are 2 to 5 cm in size. Multiple tumors are associated with a worse prognosis.[10]

PATHOPHYSIOLOGY AND MOLECULAR GENETICS

The evolution of ADC of the esophagus involves earlier losses of the p16 and p53 genes and later losses of the APC gene.[11] Aneuploidy occurs early and can be found before cancer occurs.

A multistep process has been proposed for GC starting with chronic gastritis to atrophic gastritis, intestinal metaplasia, and dysplasia before resulting in intestinal-type GC.[12] Premalignant counterparts are not seen in diffuse-type cancers.

H pylori

H pylori is implicated with atrophic gastritis, intestinal metaplasia, and dysplasia leading to intestinal type GC.[13,14] A positive association is demonstrated in regions where high-risk CagA (+) *H pylori* strains are endemic.[15] Bacterial virulence factors contributing to GC risk include vacA, babA2, OipA, and CagA.[16] Single-nucleotide polymorphisms in IL-1β and endogenous receptor antagonists (IL-1RN) are associated with increased susceptibility to *H pylori*–induced GC.[17,18]

Chromosomal Instability

Intestinal-type GC show copy number gains at 8q, 17q, and 20q and losses at 3p and 5q.[19,20] Diffuse-type GC show copy number gains at 12q and 13q and losses at 4q, 15q, 16q, and 17p.[20–22]

Microsatellite Instability

Microsatellite instability (MSI) is observed in 8% to 39% of GC.[23–28] Most studies have shown that MSI is associated with less aggressive behavior and favorable survival, whereas others indicated no prognostic impact.[29]

Microsatellite-unstable GC are associated with older age, female gender, expanding growth pattern, antral location, intestinal-type histology, a lower incidence of lymph node metastasis, and favorable prognosis. Hypermethylation of MLH1 promoter is associated with the development of sporadic GC with MSI[30,31] and is detected in 20% to 30% of nondiffuse, distal GC.

Vascular Endothelial Growth Factor

In GC, vascular endothelial growth factor (VEGF) expression is associated with advanced stage and poor survival.[32] Plasma VEGF-A and tumor neuropilin-1 are strong biomarker candidates for predicting clinical outcome in patients with advanced GC treated with VEGF inhibitor, bevacizumab.[33]

HER-2

HER-2 has been shown to be overexpressed/amplified in 6% to 35% of gastric tumors.[34–38] This overexpression/amplification is associated with GEJ tumors more than with gastric tumors.[39] Twenty percent of intestinal-type cancers have HER-2 overexpression/amplification compared with 5% of diffuse-type cancers. In the ToGA study, the addition of trastuzumab, a monoclonal antibody targeting HER-2, to palliative chemotherapy led to an overall survival benefit specifically in patients with HER-2 overexpression or amplification.[40] Trastuzumab-based combination therapy is now the standard treatment for patients with HER-2 amplified GC.

HER-2 testing
To date, HER-2 is the only validated therapeutic target in GC. The guidelines for HER2 testing of gastric or GEJ tumors were established by the ToGA trial.

Immunohistochemistry and fluorescence in situ hybridization
HER2 expression may be assessed by immunohistochemistry (IHC), with scoring ranging from 0 to 3+, or by gene amplification using fluorescence in situ hybridization (FISH) or silver in situ hybridization (SISH). The survival benefit associated with trastuzumab is seen greatest in IHC 3+ or IHC 2+ and FISH-positive patients with high HER-2 expressing tumors.

Because of the heterogeneous nature of HER-2 overexpression/amplification in GC, and because gastric tumor cells may only show HER-2 staining at the basolateral or lateral membrane regions, complete membranous staining is not a prerequisite for IHC 2+ or IHC 3+ scores in GC as it is for breast cancer.[41]

A 10% cutoff of positive cells is defined for assessment of both breast and gastric cancer. However, small biopsy specimens or tumor cell clusters are assessed regardless of the percentage of the cells staining.[41]

It should be noted that for gastric or GEJ cancers, the presence of more than 4 copies of the HER2 gene per tumor cell (if no chromosome 17 control is used) is not a positive result, a difference from breast cancer guidelines.[41]

SISH
SISH is a bright-field technique and allows the pathologist to assess tumor histology and phenotype simultaneously.[42] The concordance between SISH and FISH has been found to be greater than 95%.[43]

The guidelines for SISH positivity are the same as for FISH in gastric cancer. The National Comprehensive Cancer Network guidelines recommend that 8 to 10 biopsies be taken to allow adequate histologic interpretation of GC.[44]

The European Medical Agency recommends that specimens scoring IHC 2+ should be retested by FISH or SISH. For a HER-2:chromosome 17 ratio greater than 2, patients are eligible for trastuzumab therapy.[42]

Other Abnormalities

Cadherin 1 or E-cadherin (CDH1) is involved in the initiation and progression of both sporadic and hereditary forms of GC.[45,46] Serum soluble CDH1 is a prognostic marker for GC, and a high concentration predicts extensive tumor invasion.[47] Cyclin E gene is amplified in 15% to 20% of GC and this overexpression of cyclin E correlates with the aggressiveness of the cancer. Reduced p27 expression is a negative prognostic factor for patients with a cyclin E-positive tumor.[48] Reduced expression of retinoblastoma is associated with worse overall survival.[29] Abnormal expression of p53 significantly affects cumulative survival and p53 status may also influence response to chemotherapy.[49,50] Protection of telomeres (POT1) expression levels are significantly higher in GC of advanced stage.

TREATMENT

The treatment of EC is esophagectomy, which carries a high morbidity.[6] Surgical resection is the mainstay of treatment of early-stage GC. The prognosis for patients with advanced stage GC and GEJ cancers is poor despite new treatment strategies.[51,52] HER-2-overexpressing tumors are eligible for HER-2-targeted therapies including monoclonal antibodies (ie, Trastuzumab) or tyrosine kinase inhibitors (Lapatinib).[41] Trastuzumab-based combination therapy is now the standard treatment for patients with HER-2 amplified GC.[32]

MORPHOLOGY

Two main histologic subtypes of EC include squamous cell carcinoma and ADC. According to the World Health Organization and the Laurén classifications, 2 main histologic types of GC include the diffuse and intestinal subtypes.[53–55] The reader is referred to gastrointestinal pathology literature for further reading.[10,56]

REFERENCES

1. de Vries AC, Haringsma J, Kuipers EJ. The detection, surveillance and treatment of premalignant gastric lesions related to Helicobacter pylori infection. Helicobacter 2007;12:1–15.
2. Garcia-Gonzalez MA, Lanas A, Quintero E, et al. Gastric cancer susceptibility is not linked to pro- and anti-inflammatory cytokine gene polymorphisms in whites: a Nationwide Multicenter Study in Spain. Am J Gastroenterol 2007; 102:1878–92.
3. Rad R, Prinz C, Neu B, et al. Synergistic effect of Helicobacter pylori virulence factors and interleukin-1 polymorphisms for the development of severe histological changes in the gastric mucosa. J Infect Dis 2003;188:272–81.
4. Machado JC, Pharoah P, Sousa S, et al. Interleukin 1B and interleukin 1RN polymorphisms are associated with increased risk of gastric carcinoma. Gastroenterology 2001;121:823–9.

5. Forman D, Newell DG, Fullerton F, et al. Association between infection with Helicobacter pylori and risk of gastric cancer: evidence from a prospective investigation. BMJ 1991;302:1302–5.

6. Holmes RS, Vaughan TL. Epidemiology and pathogenesis of esophageal cancer [review]. Semin Radiat Oncol 2007;17(1):2–9.

7. Montgomery E, Goldblum JR, Greenson JK, et al. Dysplasia as a predictive marker for invasive carcinoma in Barrett esophagus: a follow-up study based on 138 cases from a diagnostic variability study. Hum Pathol 2001;32(4):379–88.

8. Siegel R, Ward E, Brawley O, et al. Cancer statistics, 2011: the impact of eliminating socioeconomic and racial disparities on premature cancer deaths. CA Cancer J Clin 2011;61(4):212–36.

9. Strong VE, Song KY, Park CH, et al. Comparison of gastric cancer survival following R0 resection in the United States and Korea using an internationally validated nomogram. Ann Surg 2010;251(4):640–6.

10. Lauwers GY. Epithelial neoplasms of the stomach. In: Odze RD, Goldblum JR, editors. Surgical pathology of the GI tract, liver, biliary tract and pancreas. Philadelphia, PA: Saunders Elsevier; 2009. p. 563–79.

11. Maley CC, Galipeau PC, Finley JC, et al. Genetic clonal diversity predicts progression to esophageal adenocarcinoma. Nat Genet 2006;38(4):468–73.

12. Correa P. Helicobacter pylori and gastric carcinogenesis. Am J Surg Pathol 1995;19(Suppl 1):S37–43.

13. Correa P. Human gastric carcinogenesis: a multistep and multifactorial process–First American Cancer Society Award Lecture on Cancer Epidemiology and Prevention. Cancer Res 1992;52(24):6735–40.

14. Correa P, Haenszel W, Cuello C, et al. A model for gastric cancer epidemiology. Lancet 1975;2(7924):58–60.

15. Cavaleiro-Pinto M, Peleteiro B, Lunet N, et al. Helicobacter pylori infection and gastric cardia cancer: systematic review and meta-analysis. Cancer Causes Control 2011;22(3):375–87.

16. Tan IB, Ng I, Tai WM, et al. Understanding the genetic basis of gastric cancer: recent advances. Expert Rev Gastroenterol Hepatol 2012;6(3):335–41.

17. El-Omar EM, Carrington M, Chow WH, et al. Interleukin-1 polymorphisms associated with increased risk of gastric cancer. Nature 2000;404(6776):398–402.

18. Persson C, Canedo P, Machado JC, et al. Polymorphisms in inflammatory response genes and their association with gastric cancer: a HuGE systematic review and meta-analyses. Am J Epidemiol 2011;173(3):259–70.

19. Kokkola A, Monni O, Puolakkainen P, et al. 17q12-21 amplicon, a novel recurrent genetic change in intestinal type of gastric carcinoma: a comparative genomic hybridization study. Genes Chromosomes Cancer 1997;20(1):38–43.

20. Wu MS, Chang MC, Huang SP, et al. Correlation of histologic subtypes and replication error phenotype with comparative genomic hybridization in gastric cancer. Genes Chromosomes Cancer 2001;30(1):80–6.

21. Weiss MM, Kuipers EJ, Postma C, et al. Genomic alterations in primary gastric adenocarcinomas correlate with clinicopathological characteristics and survival. Cell Oncol 2004;26(5–6):307–17.

22. Tsukamoto Y, Uchida T, Karnan S, et al. Genome-wide analysis of DNA copy number alterations and gene expression in gastric cancer. J Pathol 2008;216(4):471–82.

23. Han HJ, Yanagisawa A, Kato Y, et al. Genetic instability in pancreatic cancer and poorly differentiated type of gastric cancer. Cancer Res 1993;53:5087–9.

24. Lee HS, Choi SI, Lee HK, et al. Distinct clinical features and outcomes of gastric cancers with microsatellite instability. Mod Pathol 2002;15(6):632–40.

25. Beghelli S, de Manzoni G, Barbi S, et al. Microsatellite instability in gastric cancer is associated with better prognosis in only stage II cancers. Surgery 2006; 139(3):347–56.

26. Seo HM, Chang YS, Joo SH, et al. Clinicopathologic characteristics and outcomes of gastric cancers with the MSI-H phenotype. J Surg Oncol 2009; 99(3):143–7.

27. Corso G, Pedrazzani C, Marrelli D, et al. Correlation of microsatellite instability at multiple loci with long-term survival in advanced gastric carcinoma. Arch Surg 2009;144(8):722–7.

28. Gu M, Kim D, Bae Y, et al. Analysis of microsatelliteinstability, protein expression and methylation status of hMLH1 and hMSH2 genes in gastric carcinomas. Hepatogastroenterology 2009;56(91–92):899–904.

29. Yasui W, Oue N, Aung PP, et al. Molecular-pathological prognostic factors of gastric cancer: a review. Gastric Cancer 2005;8(2):86–94.

30. Nakajima T, Akiyama Y, Shiraishi J, et al. Age-related hypermethylation of the hMLH1 promoter in gastric cancers. Int J Cancer 2001;94(2):208–11.

31. Guo RJ, Arai H, Kitayama Y, et al. Microsatellite instability of papillary subtype of human gastric adenocarcinoma and hMLH1 promoter hypermethylation in the surrounding mucosa. Pathol Int 2001;51(4):240–7.

32. Janjigian YY, Kelsen DP. Genomic dysregulation in gastric tumors. J Surg Oncol 2013;107(3):237–42.

33. Van Cutsem E, de Haas S, Kang YK, et al. Bevacizumab in combination with chemotherapy as first-line therapy in advanced gastric cancer: a biomarker evaluation from the AVAGAST randomized phase III trial. J Clin Oncol 2012; 30(17):2119–27.

34. Gravalos C, Jimeno A. HER2 in gastric cancer: a new prognostic factor and a novel therapeutic target. Ann Oncol 2008;19(9):1523–9.

35. Beltran Gárate B, Yabar Berrocal A. HER2 expression in gastric cancer in Peru. Rev Gastroenterol Peru 2010;30(4):324–7 [in Spanish].

36. Hofmann M, Stoss O, Shi D, et al. Assessment of a HER2 scoring system for gastric cancer: results from a validation study. Histopathology 2008;52(7): 797–805.

37. Im SA, Kim JW, Kim JS, et al. Clinicopathologic characteristics of patients with stage III/IV (M(0)) advanced gastric cancer, according to HER2 status assessed by immunohistochemistry and fluorescence in situ hybridization. Diagn Mol Pathol 2011;20(2):94–100.

38. Tanner M, Hollmén M, Junttila TT, et al. Amplification of HER-2 in gastric carcinoma: association with Topoisomerase II alpha gene amplification, intestinal type, poor prognosis and sensitivity to trastuzumab. Ann Oncol 2005;16(2): 273–8.

39. Albarello L, Pecciarini L, Doglioni C. HER2 testing in gastric cancer. Adv Anat Pathol 2011;18(1):53–9.

40. Bang YJ, Van Cutsem E, Feyereislova A, et al. ToGA Trial Investigators. Trastuzumab in combination with chemotherapy versus chemotherapy alone for treatment of HER2-positive advanced gastric or gastro-oesophageal junction cancer (ToGA): a phase 3, open-label, randomised controlled trial. Lancet 2010; 376(9742):687–97.

41. Bang YJ. Advances in the management of HER2-positive advanced gastric and gastroesophageal junction cancer. J Clin Gastroenterol 2012;46(8):637–48.

42. Herceptin summary of product characteristics. Available at: http://www.ema. europa.eu/docs/en_GB/document_library/EPAR_Product_Information/human/ 000278/WC500074922.pdf. Accessed September 22, 2011.

43. Powell WC, Zielinski D, Ranger-Moore J, et al. Determining the HER2 status in gastric cancer: a method comparison study of two patient cohorts. ASCO Gastrointestinal Cancers Symposium. Orlando, January 22–24, 2010 [abstract 17].

44. NCCN clinical practice guidelines in oncology (NCCN guidelines). Gastric Cancer. Version 2.2011. Available at: http://www.nccn.org/professionals/physician_ gls/pdf/gastric.pdf. Accessed September 22, 2011.

45. Birchmeier W, Behrens J. Cadherin expression in carcinomas: role in the formation of cell junctions and the prevention of invasiveness. Biochim Biophys Acta 1994;1198(1):11–26.

46. Christofori G, Semb H. The role of the cell-adhesion molecule E-cadherin as a tumour-suppressor gene. Trends Biochem Sci 1999;24(2):73–6.

47. Chan AO, Lam SK, Chu KM, et al. Soluble E-cadherin is a valid prognostic marker in gastric carcinoma. Gut 2001;48(6):808–11.

48. Xiangming C, Natsugoe S, Takao S, et al. The cooperative role of p27 with cyclin E in the prognosis of advanced gastric carcinoma. Cancer 2000;89(6):1214–9.

49. Fondevila C, Metges JP, Fuster J, et al. p53 and VEGF expression are independent predictors of tumor recurrence and survival following curative resection of gastric cancer. Br J Cancer 2004;90(1):206–15.

50. Pinto-de-Sousa J, Silva F, David L, et al. Clinicopathological significance and survival influence of p53 protein expression in gastric carcinoma. Histopathology 2004;44(4):323–31.

51. Cunningham D, Allum WH, Stenning SP, et al, MAGIC Trial Participants. Perioperative chemotherapy versus surgery alone for resectable gastroesophageal cancer. N Engl J Med 2006;355(1):11–20.

52. Macdonald JS, Smalley SR, Benedetti J, et al. Chemoradiotherapy after surgery compared with surgery alone for adenocarcinoma of the stomach or gastroesophageal junction. N Engl J Med 2001;345(10):725–30.

53. Milne AN, Carneiro F, O'Morain C, et al. Nature meets nurture: molecular genetics of gastric cancer. Hum Genet 2009;126(5):615–28. http://dx.doi.org/10. 1007/s00439-009-0722-x.

54. Lauren P. The two histological main types of gastric carcinoma: diffuse and so-called intestinal-type carcinoma. An attempt at a histo- clinical classification. Acta Pathol Microbiol Scand 1965;64:31–49.

55. Hudler P. Genetic aspects of gastric cancer instability. ScientificWorldJournal 2012;2012:761909.

56. Glickman JN. Epithelial neoplasms of the esophagus. In: Odze RD, Goldblum JR, editors. Surgical pathology of the GI tract, liver, biliary tract and pancreas. Philadelphia, PA: Saunders Elsevier; 2009. p. 535–62.

Molecular Diagnostics in the Neoplasms of the Pancreas, Liver, Gall Bladder, and Extrahepatic Biliary Tract

Michael Weindel, MD[a], Muhammad Zulfiqar, MD[b],*,
Amarpreet Bhalla, MBBS, MD[c], Vinod B. Shidham, MD, FRCPath, FIAC[d]

KEYWORDS

- Pancreatic neoplasms • Liver neoplasms • Gall bladder adenoma
- Gall bladder adenocarcinoma • Molecular diagnostics • Extrahepatic biliary tract

KEY POINTS

- Pancreatic neoplasms, including ductal adenocarcinoma, solid pseudopapillary neoplasm, pancreatic endocrine neoplasms, acinar cell carcinoma and ampullary carcinoma are associated with different genetic abnormalities.
- Liver neoplasms, including hepatic adenomas, hepatocellular carcinomas, and cholangiocarcinomas, are associated with identifiable risk factors and genetic changes.
- Gall bladder adenomas and adenocarcinomas arise from distinct molecular pathways.
- The molecular abnormalities seen in these tumors are not used routinely in the molecular diagnostic laboratory.

PANCREATIC NEOPLASMS
Epidemiology

Pancreatic cancer is the fifth most common cause of cancer-related death in the United States, with an estimated incidence of 43,920 cases and 37,390 deaths in

[a] Department of Pathology, Detroit Medical Center, Karmanos Cancer Center, Wayne State University School of Medicine, 540 East Canfield, Detroit, MI 48201, USA; [b] Department of Pathology and Laboratory Medicine, Indiana University School of Medicine, 350 West 11th Street, Indianapolis, IN 46202-3082, USA; [c] PGY-3 Detroit Medical Center (WSU SOM), Pathology Department, Harper University Hospital, Detroit Medical Center, 3990 John R Street, Detroit, MI 48201, USA; [d] Deptartment of Pathology, Detroit Medical Center, Karmanos Cancer Center, Wayne State University School of Medicine, Old Hutzel Hospital (Dept of Cytology- Ground Floor), 4707 Street Antoine Boulevard, Detroit, MI 48201, USA
* Corresponding author.
E-mail addresses: mzulfiqa@iupui.edu; mizulfiqar@gmail.com

Clin Lab Med 33 (2013) 875–880
http://dx.doi.org/10.1016/j.cll.2013.08.002
0272-2712/13/$ – see front matter © 2013 Elsevier Inc. All rights reserved.

the United States in 2012.[1] Chronic pancreatitis and diabetes mellitus have been consistently related to pancreatic cancer. Other risk factors include physical inactivity, aspirin use, occupational exposure to pesticides, and dietary factors, such as carbohydrate and sugar intake.

Clinical Features

Patients present with anorexia, malaise, nausea, fatigue, and midepigastric or back pain. Significant weight loss is a characteristic feature of pancreatic cancer. Malabsorption with diarrhea and malodorous, greasy stools may also be present.[2]

Pathophysiology and Molecular Genetics

Ductal adenocarcinoma

The most common genetic changes seen in ductal adenocarcinoma seen in decreasing order of frequency include KRAS codon 12 mutations seen in 90%, loss of Smad4 (DPC4) in 55%,[3,4] and TP53 mutations seen in 50% of cases.[5] Alterations in pancreatic intraepithelial neoplasias include KRAS (early stages), p16 (middle), and DPC4 and p53 (later stages).[6,7] Intraductal papillary mucinous neoplasms (IPMNs) show molecular alterations similar to that of ductal adenocarcinoma; mutations in KRAS and TP53 are not as frequent as they are in ductal adenocarcinoma.[8] Loss of Smad4 within IPMN was the best marker for the presence of invasive carcinoma. DPC4 mutations are rarely seen in IPMNs compared with ductal adenocarcinoma.[9]

Other pancreatic neoplasms

Acinar cell carcinoma shows a lack of KRAS, TP53, and p16 alterations.[10] Well-differentiated pancreatic endocrine neoplasms (PENs) show multiple endocrine neoplasm type 1 (MEN1) mutations in approximately 20% of cases.[11–14] Hereditary cases are dominantly inherited and show loss of MEN1 gene.[5] Solid pseudopapillary neoplasms show nuclear accumulation of beta-catenin in 95%, activating beta-catenin mutation in 90%, cyclin D1 in 74%, and overexpression of p53 in 15.8% of cases.[15] Ampullary adenocarcinoma is biologically similar to ductal adenocarcinoma of the pancreas, with similar mutation frequencies of KRAS, p53, p16, and DPC4 genes.[16] KRAS mutations seem to be an early event in ampullary carcinoma pathogenesis, but their presence does not significantly correlate with survival.[17] In the setting of familial adenomatous polyposis (FAP), 64% have APC mutations, whereas 17% of sporadic tumors have APC mutations.[18]

Treatment

Gemcitabine has been the mainstay of systemic treatment for pancreatic cancer, with a modest therapeutic benefit.[19] For pancreatic endocrine neoplasms (PEN), first line therapy generally consists of a somatostatin analogue, such as octreotide. Recent studies have identified new chemotherapy combinations, such as capecitabine and temozolomide. Streptozocin in combination with either 5-fluorouracil or doxorubicin is also effective.

LIVER NEOPLASMS
Hepatic Adenoma

Epidemiology

Hepatic adenomas arise in women of childbearing age, with long-term contraceptive use as a risk factor.

Pathophysiology and molecular genetics

Hepatic adenoma is divided into 4 groups according to molecular genetic abnormalities:

Group 1: hepatocyte nuclear factor 1 alpha mutations, either somatic or germline steatosis; younger patients, diabetes, history of FAP.[20]

Group 2: beta-catenin mutations; men; mild cytologic abnormalities; focal acinar pattern; relatively less steatosis; more frequently associated with development of hepatocellular carcinoma (HCC).[20]

Group 3: formerly referred to as *telangiectatic focal nodular hyperplasia*; monoclonality; angiopoietin1-to-angiopoietin2 mRNA ratio similar to that of hepatic adenomas.[21–23]

Group 4: cases that do not fit into groups 1 through 3.

HCC

Epidemiology

HCC usually develops in the setting of chronic liver disease, particularly in patients with chronic hepatitis B and C.

Pathophysiology and molecular genetics

Molecular abnormalities noted using comparative genomic hybridization technology included gains in 8q, 1q, 17q, 12q, 20q, 5p, 6q, and Xq. The possible genes implicated include MYC (8q), MDM2 (12q), SSTR2 or GHq (17q), and MYBL2 or PTPN1 (20q). Frequent losses were also noted on 8p, 16q, 4q, 13q, 1p, 4p, 16p, 18q, 14q, 17p, 9p, and 9q. Possible genes implicated include PCDH7 (4p), FEZ1 (8p), RB1 (13q), TSHR (14q), GSPT1 (16p), CDH1 (16q), TP53 (17p), and DPC4 (18q).

Cholangiocarcinoma

Epidemiology

Cholangiocarcinoma is the second most common primary hepatic neoplasm, and its incidence has increased within the past 3 decades. Worldwide, the average age at presentation is 50 years, with the highest prevalence seen in Southeast Asia. Although several risk factors have been identified, including primary sclerosing cholangitis and chronic biliary tract inflammation, most patients with cholangiocarcinoma have no identifiable risk factors.

Pathophysiology and molecular genetics

Downregulation of beta-catenin, seen in high-grade tumors, correlates with reduced immunohistochemical staining.[24,25] Decreased p27 is associated with more aggressive tumor behavior and increased risk of vascular invasion.[26] Downregulation of BCL2 is also associated with more aggressive tumors.[27]

Clinical features

Patients with hepatic adenomas present with right upper quadrant pain. Cholangiocarcinomas become symptomatic when the tumor obstructs the biliary system, causing painless jaundice, pruritus, right upper quadrant abdominal pain, weight loss, and fever.

Molecular diagnostics

Although the described genetic changes can lead to detectable phenotypic changes, the diagnostic or prognostic usefulness of these developments is unclear, and molecular profiling does not yet have an established clinical role in patients with cholangiocarcinoma.

Treatment

Hepatic adenomas are treated with resection. The only curative therapy for HCC is surgical resection or liver transplantation. For advanced-stage disease, survival remains limited. Newer targeted therapies are being developed with increasing understanding of the molecular mechanisms of disease.

GALL BLADDER AND EXTRAHEPATIC BILIARY TRACT NEOPLASMS

Epidemiology

Gall bladder carcinoma, the most frequent malignancy of the biliary tract, has a female predominance. The mean age at diagnosis is 72 years. Gallstones and inflammation are responsible for most biliary tract abnormalities.[28]

Pathophysiology and Molecular Genetics

Adenoma

Alterations in adenomas are distinct from those observed in conventional dysplasia-carcinoma sequence of the gall bladder.[5] Bata-catenin mutations are detected in 58% of adenomas, and are rare in invasive cancer.[29] TP53 mutations are rare in adenomas but are common in flat dysplasia and invasive carcinoma. KRAS mutations are detected in approximately 25% of adenomas.[30]

Dysplasia/carcinoma in situ

Loss of heterozygosity (LOH) of 5q is an early change, and LOH of 3p and 9p is related to progression of gall bladder carcinoma. LOH of 13q and 18q is likely to be a late event.[30] Decreased FHIT (Fragile Histidine Triad) and LOH occurred at higher frequencies with increasing severity of histologic changes.[31]

Adenocarcinoma

Data support the hypothesis that adenomas and carcinomas of the gall bladder arise from distinct molecular pathways. Protein p53 overexpression is detected in approximately 50% of cases, with the highest frequency in distal common bile duct tumors.[32] KRAS and DPC4 mutations increase in frequency from low in proximal to high in distal bile duct tumors, and lower than in pancreatic tumors.[33,34] Her-2n/neu (c-erB2) amplification is noted in 70% of biliary cancers with no known correlation with prognosis.[5] Data suggests that methylation is a frequent event in cholangiocarcinomas; methylation status of the markers mentioned earlier may serve as a prognostic marker. Overall survival was poorer in patients with CpG island methylation of APC, p16, and TIMP3 than in those without methylation.

Clinical features

Gall bladder adenomas produce symptoms when they are multiple, large, or detached. Adenomas of the extrahepatic biliary tract are usually discovered incidentally or patients may present with symptoms of obstruction.[5] Advanced-stage gall bladder carcinoma presents with right upper quadrant pain, weight loss, and anorexia, but for early-stage tumors, symptoms at presentation can mimic those of chronic cholecystitis. Jaundice is not common at presentation.

SUMMARY

Although the described genetic changes in the neoplasms of the pancreas, liver, gall bladder, and extrahepatic biliary tract lead to detectable phenotypic changes, their diagnostic and prognostic usefulness is unclear and they are not used routinely in the molecular diagnostic laboratory.

REFERENCES

1. Cancer Facts and Figures 2012. Available at: http://www.cancer.org/acs/groups/content/@epidemiologysurveilance/documents/document/acspc-031941.pdf. Accessed September 7, 2013.
2. Dragovich T, Harris JE. Pancreatic cancer clinical presentation, MedScape Reference Web site. Available at: http://emedicine.medscape.com/article/280605-clinical. Accessed September 7, 2013.
3. Iacobuzio-Donahue CA, Song J, Parmiagiani G, et al. Missense mutations of MADH4: characterization of the mutational hot spot and functional consequences in human tumors. Clin Cancer Res 2004;10(5):1597–604.
4. Wilentz RE, Su GH, Dai JL, et al. Immunohistochemical labeling for dpc4 mirrors genetic status in pancreatic adenocarcinomas: a new marker of DPC4 inactivation. Am J Pathol 2000;156(1):37–43.
5. Odze RD, Goldblum JR. Surgical pathology of the GI tract, liver, biliary tract, and pancreas. Philadelphia: Saunders/Elsevier; 2009.
6. Lemoine NR, Jain S, Hughes CM, et al. Ki-ras oncogene activation in preinvasive pancreatic cancer. Gastroenterology 1992;102(1):230–6.
7. Moskaluk CA, Hruban RH, Kern SE. p16 and K-ras gene mutations in the intraductal precursors of human pancreatic adenocarcinoma. Cancer Res 1997; 57(11):2140–3.
8. Biankin AV, Biankin SA, Kench JG, et al. Aberrant p16(INK4A) and DPC4/Smad4 expression in intraductal papillary mucinous tumours of the pancreas is associated with invasive ductal adenocarcinoma. Gut 2002;50(6):861–8.
9. Iacobuzio-Donahue CA, Klimstra DS, Adsay NV, et al. Dpc-4 protein is expressed in virtually all human intraductal papillary mucinous neoplasms of the pancreas: comparison with conventional ductal adenocarcinomas. Am J Pathol 2000; 157(3):755–61.
10. Hoorens A, Lemoine NR, McLellan E, et al. Pancreatic acinar cell carcinoma. An analysis of cell lineage markers, p53 expression, and Ki-ras mutation. Am J Pathol 1993;143(3):685–98.
11. Görtz B, Roth J, Krähenmann A, et al. Mutations and allelic deletions of the MEN1 gene are associated with a subset of sporadic endocrine pancreatic and neuroendocrine tumors and not restricted to foregut neoplasms. Am J Pathol 1999; 154(2):429–36.
12. Hessman O, Lindberg D, Einarsson A, et al. Genetic alterations on 3p, 11q13, and 18q in nonfamilial and MEN 1-associated pancreatic endocrine tumors. Genes Chromosomes Cancer 1999;26(3):258–64.
13. Komminoth P. Review: multiple endocrine neoplasia type 1, sporadic neuroendocrine tumors, and MENIN. Diagn Mol Pathol 1999;8(3):107–12.
14. Moore PS, Missiaglia E, Antonello D, et al. Role of disease-causing genes in sporadic pancreatic endocrine tumors: MEN1 and VHL. Genes Chromosomes Cancer 2001;32(2):177–81.
15. Abraham SC, Klimstra DS, Wilentz RE, et al. Solid-pseudopapillary tumors of the pancreas are genetically distinct from pancreatic ductal adenocarcinomas and almost always harbor beta-catenin mutations. Am J Pathol 2002;160(4):1361–9.
16. Moore PS, Orlandini S, Zamboni G, et al. Pancreatic tumours: molecular pathways implicated in ductal cancer are involved in ampullary but not in exocrine nonductal or endocrine tumorigenesis. Br J Cancer 2001;84(2):253–62.
17. Howe JR, Klimstra DS, Cordon-Cardo C, et al. K-ras mutation in adenomas and carcinomas of the ampulla of vater. Clin Cancer Res 1997;3(1):129–33.

18. Achille A, Scupoli MT, Magalini AR, et al. APC gene mutations and allelic losses in sporadic ampullary tumours: evidence of genetic difference from tumours associated with familial adenomatous polyposis. Int J Cancer 1996;68(3):305–12.
19. Bayraktar S, Rocha Lima CM. Emerging cell-cycle inhibitors for pancreatic cancer therapy. Expert Opin Emerg Drugs 2012;17(4):571–82.
20. Zucman-Rossi J, Jeannot E, Nhieu JT, et al. Genotype-phenotype correlation in hepatocellular adenoma: new classification and relationship with HCC. Hepatology 2006;43(3):515–24.
21. Bioulac-Sage P, Rebouissou S, Sa Cunha A, et al. Clinical, morphologic, and molecular features defining so-called telangiectatic focal nodular hyperplasias of the liver. Gastroenterology 2005;128(5):1211–8.
22. Paradis V, Benzekri A, Dargère D, et al. Telangiectatic focal nodular hyperplasia: a variant of hepatocellular adenoma. Gastroenterology 2004;126(5):1323–9.
23. Paradis V, Bièche I, Dargère D, et al. A quantitative gene expression study suggests a role for angiopoietins in focal nodular hyperplasia. Gastroenterology 2003;124(3):651–9.
24. Sugimachi K, Taguchi K, Aishima S, et al. Altered expression of beta-catenin without genetic mutation in intrahepatic cholangiocarcinoma. Mod Pathol 2001; 14(9):900–5.
25. Ashida K, Terada T, Kitamura Y, et al. Expression of E-cadherin, alpha-catenin, beta-catenin, and CD44 (standard and variant isoforms) in human cholangiocarcinoma: an immunohistochemical study. Hepatology 1998;27(4):974–82.
26. Taguchi K, Aishima S, Asayama Y, et al. The role of p27kip1 protein expression on the biological behavior of intrahepatic cholangiocarcinoma. Hepatology 2001; 33(5):1118–23.
27. Ito Y, Takeda T, Sasaki Y, et al. Bcl-2 expression in cholangiocellular carcinoma is inversely correlated with biologically aggressive phenotypes. Oncology 2000; 59(1):63–7.
28. Volkan Adsay N, Klimstra DS. Benign and malignant tumors of the gallbladder and extrahepatic biliary tract. In: Odze RD, Goldblum JR, editors. Surgical pathology of the GI tract, liver, biliary tract and pancreas. 2nd edition. Philadelphia: Saunders/Elsevier; 2009.
29. Chang HJ, Jee CD, Kim WH. Mutation and altered expression of beta-catenin during gallbladder carcinogenesis. Am J Surg Pathol 2002;26(6):758–66.
30. Chang HJ, Kim SW, Kim YT, et al. Loss of heterozygosity in dysplasia and carcinoma of the gallbladder. Mod Pathol 1999;12(8):763–9.
31. Wistuba II, Ashfaq R, Maitra A, et al. Fragile histidine triad gene abnormalities in the pathogenesis of gallbladder carcinoma. Am J Pathol 2002;160(6):2073–9.
32. Batheja N, Suriawinata A, Saxena R, et al. Expression of p53 and PCNA in cholangiocarcinoma and primary sclerosing cholangitis. Mod Pathol 2000;13(12): 1265–8.
33. Argani P, Shaukat A, Kaushal M, et al. Differing rates of loss of DPC4 expression and of p53 overexpression among carcinomas of the proximal and distal bile ducts. Cancer 2001;91(7):1332–41.
34. Nagahashi M, Ajioka Y, Lang I, et al. Genetic changes of p53, K-ras, and microsatellite instability in gallbladder carcinoma in high-incidence areas of Japan and Hungary. World J Gastroenterol 2008;14(1):70–5.

Current Applications of Molecular Genetic Technologies to the Diagnosis and Treatment of Cutaneous Melanocytic Neoplasms

Muhammad Zulfiqar, MD[a],
Andrew David Thompson, MD, PhD, FCAP[b,c],*

KEYWORDS

- Melanoma • Spitz tumor • Uncertain malignant potential
- Fluorescense in situ hybridization • Ipilimumab • Vemurafenib • Imatinib

KEY POINTS

- Molecular genetic technologies are currently being used to aid in the diagnosis and treatment of cutaneous melanocytic neoplasms.
- Fluorescence in situ hybridization is being employed to aid in the determination of the nature of melanocytic neoplasms.
- A specific set of fluorescence in situ hybridization probes designed to help distinguish nevi from melanomas in challenging cases has been developed and commercialized.
- Though this technology shows much promise, additional experience with this technology and its wider usage have highlighted limitations and pitfalls in the current application of this technology.
- There is continued development of fluorescence in situ hybridization probes for use in the diagnosis and evaluation of the prognosis of challenging melanocytic neoplasms.
- Array comparative genomic hybridization is a more complex technology, currently in very limited clinical use, which may soon be used to aid in the diagnosis of melanocytic neoplasms.
- Monoclonal antibodies targeting the CTLA-4 antigen and novel therapeutic molecules designed to target specific mutations in BRAF and KIT are showing promising results.

[a] Department of Pathology and Laboratory Medicine, Indiana University School of Medicine, 350 West 11th Street, Indianapolis, IN 46202-3082, USA; [b] Department of Pathology, DMC Harper University Hospital, Wayne State University School of Medicine, 3990 John R, Detroit, MI 48201-2018, USA; [c] Barbara Ann Karmanos Cancer Institute, 4100 John R, Detroit, MI 48201, USA
* Corresponding author.
E-mail addresses: athompso2@dmc.org; andrew-d-thompson@hotmail.com

Clin Lab Med 33 (2013) 881–890
http://dx.doi.org/10.1016/j.cll.2013.08.008
0272-2712/13/$ – see front matter © 2013 Elsevier Inc. All rights reserved.

INTRODUCTION

Abnormalities in chromosomal copy numbers and chromosomal instability in general are well-accepted factors in oncogenesis and the progression of malignancies. In regard to benign melanocytic lesions (nevi) and malignant melanocytic lesions (melanomas), chromosomal aberrations of specific chromosomes are frequently seen in melanomas. Conversely, variations in chromosomal copy numbers are rarely seen in nevi.[1]

Most melanocytic neoplasms can be readily differentiated and separated dichotomously into nevi and melanomas to provide for prognosis and treatment.[2] There are several readily identifiable types of nevi with well-defined histopathologic characteristics. It is also becoming increasing clear that, in addition to nevi and melanomas, a third category of melanocytic lesions may exist (borderline melanocytic lesions/melanocytic lesions of low or intermediate malignant potential/melanocytomas) that are of intermediate malignant potential, demonstrating frequent metastases to lymph nodes but only showing rare progression to distant metastatic disease or death (**Table 1**).[3]

One well-recognized and widely discussed group of melanocytic lesions is the Spitzoid group of melanocytic lesions. At 1 end of the spectrum of these lesions are Spitz nevi, benign neoplasms usually seen in younger patients that are composed of large spindle-shaped and/or epithelioid melanocytes.[4] Cutaneous melanoma is rare in childhood, but there are many well-described cases of fatal melanomas in young patients, particularly after puberty.[5] Spitzoid melanomas are malignant melanocytic lesions with cytologic and architectural features similar to those seen in Spitz nevi.[3] Spitzoid melanomas are seen in all age groups and are well described as 1 type of melanoma that may develop in childhood.[3,6]

In addition to Spitz nevi and Spitzoid melanomas, a third group of Spitzoid tumors is often discussed. These atypical Spitzoid tumors (of uncertain biologic potential) demonstrate histologic features intermediate between those seen in Spitz nevi and Spitzoid melanomas. They represent one of the most difficult to classify sets of neoplasms in dermatopathology, and a lack of consensus regarding diagnosis is seen even among the most experienced dermatopathologists.[7] Multiple studies have recently shown that atypical Spitzoid tumors may behave as borderline melanocytic lesions, displaying a high incidence of lymph node metastases but a favorable outcome relative to melanoma.[7,8]

Table 1
Differential diagnosis. Categories of melanocytic neoplasms based on prognosis

Entity	Prognosis/Nature of Entity	Biologic Endpoint/Clinical Importance
Nevus	Benign	Cosmetic concern May be clinically indistinguishable from melanoma
Borderline melanocytic lesion/melanocytic lesion of low or intermediate potential/melanocytoma	Low or intermediate malignant potential	Potential for recurrence or metastasis to regional lymph nodes No or only rare progression to distant metastatic disease and death
Melanoma	Malignant	Frequent progression to distant metastasis and death

THE GENETICS OF MELANOCYTIC LESIONS

Building upon the knowledge that melanomas, unlike nevi, harbor chromosomal anomalies, several studies have demonstrated that melanomas are genetically hetero-geneous. In 2005, Bastian led a group of researchers in a fundamental study. Using genome-wide comparisons of alterations in the number of copies of DNA and ana-lyses of the mutational statuses of BRAF and RAS genes, they were able to delineate 4 genetically distinct groups of melanomas. These groups of melanomas were defined by anatomic location (acral and mucosal) and exposure to ultraviolet light (with or without chronic sun-induced damage).[9]

Studies such as that mentioned previously have brought into question the current histogenetic typing of melanomas into such categories as superficial spreading, len-tigo maligna, nodular, and acral lentiginous. These categories are not an independent prognostic factor for melanoma, and the previously mentioned study found that mel-anomas on acral skin clustered according their genetic changes regardless of their histogenetic types.[9] Finally, studies have shown that well-characterized receptors and signal transduction molecules (such as BRAF, RAS, KIT) are often mutated in some sets of melanomas but only rarely in others.[9,10]

Though most nevi do not show chromosomal abnormalities, it has been demon-strated that 15% of benign Spitz nevi show amplification of 11p.[11] This chromosomal location is where HRAS is found; HRAS mutations are seen in Spitz nevi but are not described in Spitzoid melanomas or Spitz tumors that have progressed to malig-nancy.[12] More recently, specific mutations, including mutations of the BAP1 gene on chromosome 3, have been described in atypical Spitz tumors.[13,14]

THE USE OF FLUORESCENCE IN SITU HYBRIDIZATION IN THE DIAGNOSIS OF MELANOCYTIC NEOPLASMS

For fluorescence in situ hybridization (FISH), short DNA probes are hybridized to formalin-fixed paraffin-embedded (FFPE) tissue. These probes have overlapping wavelength spectra that limit to 4 the number of probes that can be used together in a single experiment.[1] In a seminal paper, Gerami and colleagues[15] described the development of a 4-probe set to serve as an ancillary tool in the diagnosis of melano-cytic lesions. Using multiple cohorts of melanocytic lesions, this team settled on a group of 4 probes and then combined numerical cut-offs of parameters for single probes and pairs of probes to yield the best combination of sensitivity and specificity by area under the receiver operator curve. The probes and corresponding genes were 6p25 (RREB1), Centromere 6, 6q23 (MYB1), and 11q13 (CCND1). These probes and parameters were applied to a third cohort of melanocytic lesions and showed a sensi-tivity of 86.7% and a specificity of 95.4% in the differentiation of nevi from melanomas. Finally, in a critical proof of the use of this technology in cases in which it is most needed, the probes and parameters were applied to a group of 27 ambiguous mela-nocytic tumors, and all 6 of the primary tumors that had eventually metastasized were positive by this FISH assay.[15]

Using the fact that melanomas show genetic instability and nevi do not, this group conducted a study with results that are impressive. This FISH technology involving these 4 probes was patented and is being commercialized by Abbott Molecular (Des Plaines, IL) with rights having been granted to NeoGenomics Laboratories (Fort Myers, FL). Outside the United States, Abbott Molecular's assay is available as a diag-nostic kit, but in the United States, this assay is only performed at the academic centers involved in the development of the test and as a commercial service by Neo-Genomics Laboratories.[1]

In a review article from 2011, Gerami and Zembowicz chronicled and analyzed experiences of the dermatopathology community with FISH for the diagnosis of melanocytic neoplasms since the development and commercialization of this 4-probe set. They pointed out that the sensitivity and specificity mentioned previously are not satisfactory for the diagnosis of melanoma, and "thus melanoma FISH must not be used as a stand-alone test and has to be considered as a diagnostic adjunct."[1] They also highlighted that numerical FISH parameters are empirically derived and thus will vary between laboratories and need to be continually validated.[1] Like any laboratory test, the parameters can be arbitrarily changed to increase either the sensitivity or the specificity, but there will be an inevitable decrease in the specificity or sensitivity, respectively.

Gerami and Zembowicz reviewed NeoGenomics' use of the probe set and noted that NeoGenomics uses different numerical parameters (than those described in Gerami's seminal paper) and that NeoGenomics' data (from the time of the publication their review article) demonstrate only 75% sensitivity for melanoma. They also pointed out that the use of the current FISH test will result in as low as a 50% sensitivity for certain types of melanomas. They explained that for challenging and borderline melanocytic lesions (where dermatopathologists would most like a molecular assay to aid in diagnoses), there are unavoidable and fundamental difficulties in establishing the sensitivity and specificity of FISH assays.

Another review of experience with and reflections on FISH technology was provided in an editorial by McCalmont.[16] This author mentioned a sensitivity lower than 70% for the use of FISH in thin conventional melanomas. He also described an example of a putative "FISH-negative melanoma."[16] The inevitable existence of such entities is a critical point for all those reading this article and must be taken into account by all those who would interpret or use the results of a FISH analysis of a melanocytic lesion.

McCalmont and Gerami and Zembowicz highlight the critical and disappointing insight that the sensitivity of FISH is likely to be particularly low in the setting of Spitzoid lesions.[1,16] This point is also demonstrated in a paper that described a sensitivity of 70% for the standard FISH probes in unequivocal Spitzoid melanomas.[17] Another fundamental take home message from their articles is that the results of FISH assays must not be used alone. The only effective and acceptable use of the currently available FISH technology for melanocytic lesions is as an additional piece of information that is integrated with histopathologic and clinical data into a comprehensive evaluation of that lesion (**Box 1**).[1,16]

Box 1
Pitfalls. Difficulties with the use of FISH technologies in the diagnosis of melanocytic lesions

- FISH is inherently limited by only targeting certain specific chromosomes and genes.
- The sensitivity and specificity of the currently widely used FISH probe set are too low for the use of this technology as a stand-alone test.
- The parameters can be arbitrarily changed to increase either the sensitivity or the specificity, but there will be an inevitable decrease in the specificity or sensitivity respectively.
- The use of the current FISH probe set and even FISH technology in general may demonstrate particularly disappointing results in the settings of challenging and borderline melanocytic lesions (such as Spitzoid tumors).
- FISH-negative melanomas exist.
- FISH must be used in conjunction with careful histopathologic analysis and integration of clinical information.

THE NEXT ROUND OF MOLECULAR GENETIC TECHNOLOGIES FOR THE ANALYSIS OF MELANOCYTIC NEOPLASMS

Researchers continue to learn about the molecular genetics of melanocytic neoplasms while pathologists and clinicians are gleaning clinically relevant information from the initial application of FISH technology in the analysis of melanocytic lesions. What adjustments to this technology and what future technologies will very soon be getting a chance to prove their potentials in patient care? One obvious limiting facet of the current FISH technology is that chromosomal aberrations will not be identified if they do not involve the chromosomes (only chromosomes 6 and 11) that are being targeted by the set of FISH probes that is currently in use. In particular, it is clear that anomalies involving other chromosomes (including chromosomes 3 and 9) are seen in and may be more common in melanomas of childhood, Spitzoid melanomas, and atypical Spitzoid melanocytic proliferations.[13,14,16,17] Technologies being developed that will circumnavigate the current FISH assay's limitations include the use of new or additional FISH probes to elucidate the diagnosis and prognosis of these lesions as well as the inter-related but more complex technology of array comparative genomic hybridization (aCGH).

The focus of the initial FISH assay on chromosomes 6 and 11 and subsequent experience with this assay have suggested to experts the need for the development and application of additional FISH probes to aid in the diagnosis of melanocytic neoplasms.[1,16] Gerami and colleagues[18] described the development and use of a novel set of 4 FISH probes (9p21, 6q25, 11q13, and 8q24) that demonstrated a sensitivity of 94% and a specificity of 98% when applied to the final validation cohort of melanocytic neoplasms. In light of the current limitation on the number of FISH probes that can be used concurrently and the relatively poor performance of the current set of FISH probes in specific groups of challenging melanocytic neoplasms, it has been suggested that distinct FISH probe sets be developed for use in particular clinical and histopathologic contexts.[1,16] One illustration of this approach is an article highlighting the usefulness of the current 4-probe set in the specific setting of blue nevus-like melanoma.[19] Another illustration of this approach is seen in an article, cited previously, where FISH probes against 9p21 and Cep9 were used in a complementary fashion with the standard 4-FISH probe set. This combination of assays demonstrated an impressive 85% sensitivity in Spitzoid melanomas.[17]

Another recent angle of attack on the molecular analysis of melanocytic neoplasms, with obvious clinical applications, is the use of FISH probes and probe sets as prognostic tools. One study showed that copy number changes in 11q13 and 8q34 are strongly associated with melanoma prognosis and likely would complement the traditional prognostic parameters used by the American Joint Committee on Cancer (AJCC).[20] Additionally, in a particularly challenging arena, multiple studies have demonstrated that FISH probes (including 9p21, 6p25, 11q13, and 6q23) can be used to stratify the prognoses of atypical Spitzoid melanocytic neoplasms.[11,14,21]

As is clear from the previous discussion, FISH is inherently limited by only targeting certain specific chromosomes and genes. In contrast, the technique of aCGH provides for simultaneous analysis of chromosomal anomalies throughout the entire genome. There are, of course, disadvantages to aCGH, including the requirement for more tissue (relative to FISH), its inability to identify small clones of aberrant cells, and its inability to detect point mutations and balanced chromosomal translocations.[22] The greatest current disadvantage to aCGH is its cost and complexity that, for the time being, limit its use mostly to investigative studies in a small number of laboratories.[22] The promise of this technology to aid in clinical diagnoses in the not too distant future was recently hinted at by its use to detect chromosomal changes indicative of melanoma in a blue nevus-like atypical melanocytic proliferation that eventually underwent malignant transformation and led to the death of the patient (**Box 2**).[23]

THERAPEUTIC APPROACHES FOR METASTATIC MELANOMA IN THE MOLECULAR AGE

Metastatic melanoma is an aggressive malignancy. It shows poor response to single- and multiagent chemotherapy. Dacarbazine (DTIC), interleukin 2 (IL-2), and interferon-alpha (IFN) have been standard chemotherapeutic and immunotherapeutic agents for melanoma for many years, despite an absence of or limited survival advantage in clinical trials.[24] BRAF and c-kit (KIT) mutations are frequent genetic changes in metastatic melanoma.[25] Monoclonal antibodies targeting CTLA-4 and novel therapeutic molecules designed to target specific BRAF and KIT mutations are newer therapies showing promising results.

Ipilimumab (Anti-CTLA-4 Antibody)

Ipilimumab, a humanized IgG1 monoclonal antibody targeting the cytotoxic T cell-associated antigen 4 (CTLA-4), was the first drug to demonstrate an improvement in overall survival (OS) compared with the standard of care for melanoma. It augments T cell activation.[26–29] When given in combination with the glycoprotein vaccine gp 100, the antibody showed improved OS when compared with vaccine alone. In patients with previously treated metastatic melanoma, an improvement in OS was seen when ipilimumab was used in combination with chemotherapy compared with chemotherapy alone.

BRAF Mutation and Anti-BRAF Agents

Activating mutations of the gene encoding for BRAF are found in 40% to 60% of melanomas. All mutations are present within the kinase domain. A single amino acid substitution (V600E) accounts for 80% of these mutations.[30] The V600E mutation alters the 600 amino acid position on the BRAF protein from valine (GUU, GUC, GUA or GUG) to glutamic acid (GAA or GAG).[31] Additional activating mutations such as the BRAF V600K and BRAF V600R mutations have also been identified in melanomas.[30]

Zelboraf (vemurafenib)

Zelboraf (also known as PLX4032 and vemurafenib) is an orally delivered, US Food and Drug Administration (FDA)-approved drug available for the treatment of melanoma patients with the BRAF V600E mutation.[32] A large phase 2 second-line trial in 132 patients confirmed a high response rate and longer median progression

---

Box 2

Future technologies. The next round of molecular genetic technologies for the analysis of melanocytic neoplasms

- Additional FISH probe sets, especially those designed for specific clinical or histopathologic settings
- Complementary FISH probe sets used in combinations
- FISH probes as prognostic tools
- aCGH

free-survival (PFS).[33] The approval of vemurafenib was supported by an international, multicenter trial.[34]

Treatment with vemurafenib is discouraged in wild-type BRAF melanomas, because data from preclinical models have demonstrated that BRAF inhibitors can enhance rather than down-regulate the mitogen-activated protein kinase (MAPK) pathway in tumor cells with wild-type BRAF and upstream RAS mutations.[35-38]

Dabrafenib

Dabrafenib (GSK2118436) is a newer drug undergoing testing and has shown efficacy in patients with the BRAF V600E mutation.[39] When compared with dacarbazine (DTIC) in the BREAK-3 trial, dabrafenib showed longer PFS. OS data were limited by the median duration of follow-up. Partial response (PR) and complete response (CR) were also higher in patients receiving dabrafenib versus dacarbazine.

KIT Inhibitors

Unlike melanomas that occur in areas of the body with intermittent or chronic exposure to ultraviolet light, melanomas arising in non-sun-exposed areas such as the mucosal surfaces, palms, soles, and nail beds are associated with different risk factors and result from different genetic changes. For these melanoma subtypes, BRAF mutations are less common, and about one-third of these uncommon melanomas have amplifications or activating mutations of the receptor tyrosine kinase KIT.[9] Some drugs used to treat other cancers, such as imatinib and nilotinib, are known to target cells with KIT mutations. Clinical trials are now looking to see if these and other drugs might help people with particular types of melanoma. Phase 2 and 3 trials are available for patients with unresectable stage 3 or stage 4 melanoma harboring KIT mutations.

Imatinib

Imatinib was demonstrated to have a remarkable tumor response in a patient with a mutated KIT gene in a melanoma in a phase 2 study in patients with metastatic melanoma.[40] This patient had a near complete response by fluorodeoxyglucose-positron emission tomography (FDG-PET)/computed tomography (CT). However, numerous phase 2 studies using imatinib to treat unselected groups of patients with metastatic

Table 2
Treatment options. Summary of melanoma treatments discussed in this chapter

Drug	Class or Mechanism of Action
Dacarbazine (DTIC)	Chemotherapy
IL-2	Immunotherapy
IFN	Immunotherapy
Ipilimumab (anti-CTLA-4 antibody)	Humanized immunoglobulin G 1 (IgG1) monoclonal antibody targeting the cytotoxic T cell- associated antigen 4 (CTLA-4) Augments T cell activation
Zelboraf (vemurafenib, PLX4032)	Targets cells with BRAF V600E mutation
Dabrafenib (GSK2118436)	Targets cells with BRAF V600E mutation
Imatinib	Targets cells with KIT mutations
Nilotinib	Targets cells with KIT mutations (2nd generation)
Dasatinib	Targets cells with KIT mutations (2nd generation)

melanoma showed inconsistent tumor response.[41–43] Other studies have demonstrated the value of imatinib in select groups of patients with metastatic melanomas with KIT alterations.[44,45] The introduction of second-generation tyrosine kinase inhibitors, such as nilotinib and dasatinib, is expanding the interest in inhibiting mutated KIT in metastatic melanomas (**Table 2**).

REFERENCES

1. Gerami P, Zembowicz A. Update on fluorescence in situ hybridization in melanoma. Arch Pathol Lab Med 2011;135:830–7.
2. Zembowicz A, Prieto V. Melanocytic lesions: current state of knowledge—part II. Arch Pathol Lab Med 2011;135:298–9.
3. Zembowicz A, Scolyer R. Nevus/melanocytoma/melanoma. Arch Pathol Lab Med 2011;135:300–6.
4. Zedek D, McCalmont T. Spitz nevi, atypical Spitzoid neoplasms, and Spitzoid melanoma. Clin Lab Med 2011;31:311–20.
5. Paradela S, Fonseca E, Prieto V. Melanoma in children. Arch Pathol Lab Med 2011;135:307–16.
6. Paradela S, Fonseca E, Pita-Fernandez S, et al. Spitzoid and non-Spitzoid melanoma in children, a prognostic comparative study. J Eur Acad Dermatol Venereol 2013;27:1214–21. http://dx.doi.org/10.1111/j.1468-3083.
7. Ludgate M, Fullen D, Lee J, et al. The atypical Spitz tumor of uncertain biologic potential. Cancer 2009;115:631–41.
8. Sepehr A, Chao E, Trefrey B, et al. Long-term outcome of Spitz-type melanocytic tumors. Arch Dermatol 2011;147:1173–9.
9. Curtin J, Fridlyand J, Kageshita T, et al. Distinct sets of genetic alterations in melanoma. N Engl J Med 2005;353:2135–47.
10. Handolias D, Hamilton A, Salemi R, et al. Clinical responses observed with imatinib or sorafenib in melanoma patients expressing mutations in KIT. Br J Cancer 2010;102:1219–23.
11. Raskin L, Ludgate M, Iyer R, et al. Copy number variations and clinical outcome in atypical Spitz tumors. Am J Surg Pathol 2011;35:243–52.
12. van Engen-van Grunsven A, van Dijk M, Ruiter D, et al. HRAS-mutated Spitz tumors, a subtype of Spitz tumors with distinct features. Am J Surg Pathol 2010;34:1436–41.
13. Busam K, Sung J, Wiesner T, et al. Combined BRAF[V600E]-positive melanocytic lesions with large epithelioid cells lacking BAP1 expression and conventional nevomelanocytes. Am J Surg Pathol 2013;37:193–9.
14. Shen L, Cooper C, Bajaj S, et al. Atypical Spitz tumors with 6q23 deletions: a clinical, histological, and molecular study. Am J Dermatopathol 2013. http://dx.doi.org/10.1097/DAD.0b013e31828671bf. Accessed July 28, 2013.
15. Gerami P, Jewell S, Morrison L, et al. Fluorescence in situ hybridization (FISH) as an ancillary diagnostic tool in the diagnosis of melanoma. Am J Surg Pathol 2009;33:1146–56.
16. McCalmont T. Fillet of FISH. J Cutan Pathol 2011;38:327–8.
17. Gammon B, Beilfuss B, Guitart J, et al. Enhanced detection of Spitzoid melanomas using fluorescence in situ hybridization with 9p21 as an adjunctive probe. Am J Surg Pathol 2012;36:81–8.
18. Gerami P, Li G, Pouryazdanparast P, et al. A highly specific and discriminatory FISH assay for distinguishing between benign and malignant melanocytic neoplasms. Am J Surg Pathol 2012;36:808–17.

19. Pouryazdanparast P, Newman M, Mafee M, et al. Distinguishing epithelioid blue nevus from blue nevus-like melanoma using fluorescence in situ hybridization. Am J Surg Pathol 2009;33:1396–400.

20. Gerami P, Jewell S, Pouryazdanparast P, et al. Copy number gains in 11q13 and 8q34 are highly linked to prognosis in cutaneous malignant melanoma. J Mol Diagn 2011;13:352–8.

21. Gerami P, Scolyer R, Xu X, et al. Risk assessment for atypical Spitzoid melanocytic neoplasms using FISH to identify chromosomal copy number aberrations. Am J Surg Pathol 2013;37:676–84.

22. Braun-Falco M, Schempp W, Weyers W. Molecular diagnosis in dermatopathology: what makes sense, and what doesn't. Exp Dermatol 2008;18:12–23.

23. Held L, Metzler G, Eigentler T, et al. Recurrent nodules in a periauricular plaque-type blue nevus with fatal outcome. J Cutan Pathol 2012;39:1088–93.

24. Ives N, Stowe R, Lorigan P, et al. Chemotherapy compared with biochemotherapy for the treatment of metastatic melanoma: a meta-analysis of 18 trials involving 2,621 patients. J Clin Oncol 2007;253:5426–34.

25. Julia F, Thomas L, Dalle S. New therapeutical strategies in the treatment of metastatic disease. Dermatol Ther 2012;25:452–7.

26. O'Day S, Hamid O, Urba W. Targeting cytotoxic T-lymphocyte antigen-4 (CTLA-4): a novel strategy for the treatment of melanoma and other malignancies. Cancer 2007;110:2614–27.

27. Fong L, Small E. Anti-cytotoxic T-lymphocyte antigen-4 antibody: the first in an emerging class of immunomodulatory antibodies for cancer treatment. J Clin Oncol 2008;26:5275–83.

28. Robert C, Ghiringhelli F. What is the role of cytotoxic T lymphocyte-associated antigen 4 blockade in patients with metastatic melanoma? Oncologist 2009;14:848–61.

29. Hodi F, O'Day S, McDermott D, et al. Improved survival with ipilimumab in patients with metastatic melanoma. N Engl J Med 2010;363:711–23.

30. Davies H, Bignell G, Cox C, et al. Mutations of the BRAF gene in human cancer. Nature 2002;417:949–54.

31. Chapman P, Hauschild A, Robert C, et al. BRIM-3 Study Group. Improved survival with vemurafenib in melanoma with BRAF V600E mutation. N Engl J Med 2011;364:2507–16.

32. Available at: http://www.zelboraf.com. Accessed September 7, 2013.

33. Ribas A, Kim K, Schuchter L. BRIM-2: an open label, multicenter phase II study of vemurafenib in previously treated patients with BRAF V600E mutation-positive metastatic melanoma. J Clin Oncol 2011;29 [abstract: 8509].

34. A study of RO5185426 in comparison with dacarbazine in previously untreated patients with metastatic melanoma (BRIM 3). Available at: http://clinicaltrials.gov/show/NCT01006980. Accessed September 7, 2013.

35. Schwartzentruber D, Lawson D, Richards J, et al. gp100 peptide vaccine and interleukin-2 in patients with advanced melanoma. N Engl J Med 2011;364:2119–27.

36. Heidorn S, Milagre C, Whittaker S, et al. Kinase-dead BRAF and oncogenic RAS cooperate to drive tumor progression through CRAF. Cell 2010;140:209–21.

37. Hatzivassiliou G, Song K, Yen I, et al. RAF inhibitors prime wild-type RAF to activate the MAPK pathway and enhance growth. Nature 2010;464:431–5.

38. Poulikakos P, Zhang C, Bollag G, et al. RAF inhibitors transactivate RAF dimers and ERK signalling in cells with wild-type BRAF. Nature 2010;464:427–30.

39. Investigational drug, GSK2118436 (dabrafenib), reported to demonstrate clinical activity in BRAF-mutant patients with brain metastases (BREAK-MB trial). Available at: http://clinicaltrials.gov/show/NCT01266967. Accessed September 7, 2013.

40. Hodi F, Friedlander P, Corless C, et al. Major response to imatinib mesylate in KIT-mutated melanoma. J Clin Oncol 2008;26:2046–51.

41. Wyman K, Atkins M, Prieto V, et al. Multicenter phase II trial of high-dose imatinib mesylate in metastatic melanoma: significant toxicity with no clinical efficacy. Cancer 2006;106:2005–11.

42. Kim K, Eton O, Davis D, et al. Phase II trial of imatinib mesylate in patients with metastatic melanoma. Br J Cancer 2008;99:734–40.

43. Ugurel S, Hildenbrand R, Zimpfer A, et al. Lack of clinical efficacy of imatinib in metastatic melanoma. Br J Cancer 2005;92:1398–405.

44. Carvajal R, Antonescu C, Wolchok J, et al. KIT as a therapeutic target in metastatic melanoma. JAMA 2011;305:2327–34.

45. Guo J, Si L, Kong Y, et al. Phase II, open-label, single-arm trial of imatinib mesylate in patients with metastatic melanoma harboring c-Kit mutation or amplification. J Clin Oncol 2011;29:2904–9.

Breast Carcinoma
Molecular Profiling and Updates

Sudeshna Bandyopadhyay, MD*, Rouba Ali-Fehmi, MD

KEYWORDS

- Breast carcinoma • Molecular profiling • Updates • Breast cancer

KEY POINTS

- Understanding the molecular heterogeneity underlying the clinical heterogeneity of breast cancer.
- Molecular and genetic variations in breast cancer with impact on treatment and prognosis.
- Correlation of the histologic variants of breast cancer and their molecular correlates.
- Introduction to progression of in situ carcinoma to invasive carcinoma.

Breast carcinoma is the most common malignancy affecting women in the United States, comprising almost 29% of all cancers occurring in women. Moreover, it is the second most common cause of mortality, responsible for 14% of cancer-related mortality.[1] It is estimated to increase both in this country and globally.

Traditionally, this tumor is classified based on morphologic features.[2] The most common subtype is invasive ductal carcinoma, not otherwise specified (IDC-NOS). This subtype accounts for approximately 60% to 75% of all breast carcinomas. Established prognostic factors associated with survival in breast cancer are clinicopathologic factors, such as tumor size and grade, lymph node involvement, margin status, and lymph vascular invasion.[3] Predictive biologic markers that are in use clinically are estrogen and progesterone receptors and Her-2/neu receptor status. Predictive markers are used to determine subsequent treatment options and estimate the response to treatment.[4] Receptor expression is determined using validated immunohistochemical methods. In the case of Her-2/neu, fluorescence in situ hybridization assay is performed to evaluate gene amplification in the event of equivocal Her-2/neu protein expression by immunohistochemistry. The testing methodology and protocols, cutoff values, and reporting guidelines are based on the guidelines from the College of American Pathologists/American Society of Clinical Oncology.[5]

Department of Pathology, Wayne State University, 540 E Canfield Street, Detroit, MI 48201, USA
* Corresponding author.
E-mail address: SBandyop@dmc.org

Clin Lab Med 33 (2013) 891–909
http://dx.doi.org/10.1016/j.cll.2013.08.009
0272-2712/13/$ – see front matter © 2013 Elsevier Inc. All rights reserved.

labmed.theclinics.com

Over the past decades, the heterogeneity of breast carcinomas has been acknowledged and studied. Observations regarding variable outcome in patients with breast cancer have supported these theories. A landmark study by Perou and colleagues[6] illustrated that the heterogeneity of breast carcinoma was reflected in the molecular makeup of these tumors. Using cDNA technology, the investigators analyzed 65 tumors from 42 individuals, including 20 paired samples before and after chemotherapy. For the purpose of this study, 496 genes, nominated as the "intrinsic gene subset," were included for analysis. Differences in specific signaling pathways, cellular components, and proliferation gene expressions were identified as variations in expression of different subsets of genes. Using hierarchical clustering to analyze these tumors, 2 main groups of tumors were identified based on the estrogen receptor (ER) status: estrogen-positive tumors and estrogen-negative tumors (**Fig. 1**).[6–8] Estrogen-positive tumors corresponded to the luminal subtype, whereas the estrogen-negative group included the ERBB2-enriched and the basal groups.[6]

Also identified as a separate group was the normal breast subtype, which is characterized by genes normally characterizing adipose tissue and basal cell genes, with a low expression of luminal cell genes. It is thought that this group may represent contamination by the normal breast parenchyma and needs further investigation.

A subsequent study by Sorlie and colleagues[7] extended the cohort to include 38 additional tumors (total of 78 cases). From the initial gene subset, 456 genes were selected for analysis. Expanding the size of the cohort allowed for the identification of subclasses within the estrogen receptor–positive group.

Based on the aforementioned molecular studies, breast carcinomas can be classified as follows:

a. Estrogen positive
   1. Luminal A
   2. Luminal B
b. Estrogen negative
   3. Her-2/neu
   4. Triple negative
   5. Normal breast like

LUMINAL A

This subtype is characterized by the upregulation of estrogen receptor gene (ESR-1) and related genes, such as GATA 3, FOX A1, and LIV 1. Her-2/neu gene amplification is not seen. By immunohistochemistry, these tumors are characterized as estrogen receptor positive and Her-2/neu negative. They are positive for luminal cytokeratins, such as CK 8/18.

These tumors are generally well differentiated, more likely to be low stage (T1) with increased expression of progesterone receptor, low proliferation index, and negative Her-2/neu expression compared with luminal B tumors. These tumors are also associated with a significantly better recurrence-free survival and superior overall survival.[3,8–11] Additionally, the level of progesterone receptor expression seems to be a significant prognosticator in luminal A tumors whereby levels more than 20% are associated with a better survival[9] compared with luminal B tumors. In the study by Sotirou and colleagues, the 10-year relapse-free survival for luminal A tumors was 80%. Similarly, this subtype constitutes the largest group, comprising approximately 60% of all breast cancers, and also shows a lower relapse rate (9% within 5 years for this group of tumors).[3] Endocrine therapy alone is considered sufficient for this group of tumors.[12]

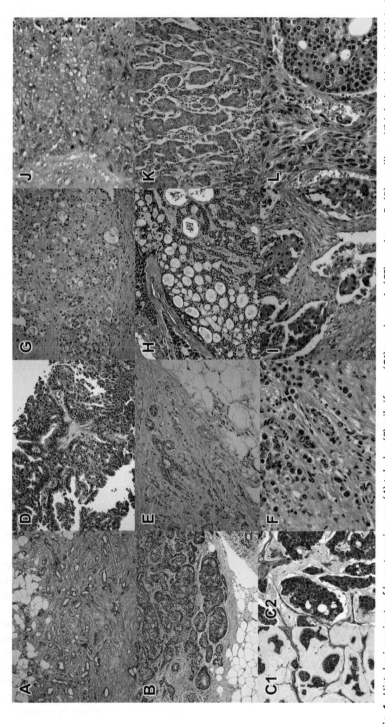

Fig. 1. Histologic variants of breast carcinoma: (A) tubular, (B) cribriform, (C1) mucinous B, (D) papillary, (E) lobular (classic), (F) lobular (pleomorphic), (G) secretory, (H) adenoid cystic, (I) apocrine, (J) atypical medullary, (K) micropapillary, (L) metaplastic (Hematoxylin & Eosin, 20×).

LUMINAL B

Increased expression for the ESR-1 and related genes, expression of luminal cytokeratins (CK 8/18), and increased expression of proliferation genes, such as CCNB1, MYBL2, and MKI67 characterize the luminal B subtype.[7] In comparison with luminal A tumors, these tumors tend to have a lower expression of the estrogen receptor–related gene set. Additionally, these tumors have higher proliferation rates, evidenced by Ki-67 nuclear labeling by immunohistochemistry, and also overexpress the ERBB2 gene, at least in a subset of cases. Therefore, luminal B tumors seem to be a more heterogeneous group and can be defined as ER +/Her-2/neu-/Ki-67 $\geq$14%.[12] Morphologically, they tend to be of a higher grade and have a worse outcome clinically with greater chances of relapse when compared with luminal A tumors.[3,10,11,13] Incorporating the Ki-67 labeling index has been reported to have significant value in stratifying the luminal tumors and identifying different subgroups with poor prognosis.[14] Although a cutoff of 14% is used to stratify risk in these tumors,[14] it is important to remember that this cutoff value does not represent a true bimodal distribution because the expression of Ki-67 is a continuum,[15] leaving this cutoff to debate and requiring further validating studies.[16,17] If left untreated, luminal B tumors have a relapse risk similar to basal-type tumors.[18] Accurately identifying these tumors is vital because treatment regimens are based on this. Additional chemotherapy and anti-Her2–related drugs are indicated in these cases.[12]

Comparative genomic hybridization (CGH) studies have shown that recurrent chromosomal changes are present within the luminal group. Concurrent deletions of 16q and gains of 1q, which are considered hallmark changes associated with low-grade ductal carcinoma, are seen in most ER-positive carcinomas, more frequent in the low-grade ER-positive disease.[19] These chromosomal alterations are rare in ER-negative tumors, suggesting that the progression from ER-positive to ER-negative disease rarely happens, if ever.

One of the most common gene mutations present in luminal breast cancers involves the PIK3CA gene. In addition to adding prognostic significance, this may be important as a therapeutic target.

ERBB2-ENRICHED (HER-2/NEU–POSITIVE) SUBTYPE

This subtype approximates 15% of all breast carcinomas. These tumors exhibit a relatively high histologic grade, affecting approximately 75% of these tumors. By genomic analysis, these tumors show increased expression of the Her-2/neu gene and other genes related to the Her-2/neu amplicon, such as GRB 7 and TRAP 100 on chromosome 17q12. Genes related to proliferation also show increased expression. By immunohistochemistry, these tumors exhibit estrogen receptor negativity and Her-2/neu protein positivity. However, it is important to understand that a substantial proportion of Her-2/neu protein–expressing tumors will belong in the luminal B subtype, and not all of these tumors will exhibit gene amplification. Mutations related to the p53 gene are seen in a significant proportion of these tumors, estimated at 40%.

Her-2/neu–positive tumors, at presentation, seem to be associated significantly with multifocal/multicentric disease, positive lymph nodes, and high-volume nodal involvement ($\geq$4 nodes) when compared with luminal A disease.[20] Clinically, these tumors behave in an aggressive fashion. However, in the recent past, the outcome of these tumors has been modified by anti-Her-2 treatments, which has had a positive impact on survival.[21,22] Additionally, these tumors reportedly show a better response to chemotherapeutic agents.[23–25] These tumors also have a better response to neoadjuvant therapy when compared with the luminal subtypes, with complete pathologic response seen in a large proportion of these tumors.[26] Local recurrences are most commonly seen with Her-2/neu–positive tumors, approximating 8.0% compared with 1.8% in luminal A tumors over a 5-year period following breast-conserving surgery.[27] Similarly, significantly lower rates of regional relapse-free survival was seen in this group (along with the basal subtype)[28] when compared with the luminal A subtype. Bone and liver metastasis is seen frequently with the Her-2/neu–positive subtype.[29]

BASAL-LIKE SUBTYPE

The basal phenotype is characterized by the lack of expression of estrogen receptors and related genes and ERBB2-related genes but show increased expression of KRT5, KRT17, CX3CL1, Annexin 8, and TRIM29. As the name implies, there is increased expression of cytokeratins related to the basal/myoepithelial cells. Also seen is an increased expression of epidermal growth factor receptor (EGFR). A large proportion of these tumors (approximately 75%) contain mutations in the p53 gene. By immuno-histochemistry, these tumors are negative for estrogen and progesterone receptors and Her-2/neu, while being positive for basal cytokeratins and EGFRs. The common basal cytokeratins used to identify these tumors are CK 5/6, CK 17, and CK 19 using immunohistochemical methods.

Morphologically, these tumors are high grade with a high mitotic rate, necrosis, pushing borders, and peritumoral lymphocytic infiltrate.[30] Clinically, these tumors present at a younger age, are more common in the African American population, and present with larger tumors with a higher proportion of concomitant lymph node metastasis (reviewed in Ref.[31]). These tumors have a poor prognosis, compared with luminal tumors, with a significantly shorter relapse-free survival and with a high proportion of women relapsing in less than 3 years. Basal tumors also have a higher proportion of metastasis to the central nervous system.[29]

For routine clinical use, surrogate immunohistochemical markers are used to classify tumors into the intrinsic subtypes (**Table 1**).[32] This classification is important because subsequent treatment decisions are based on this categorization.

More recently, additional subtypes have since been described, which are as follows.

Claudin Low Subtype

These tumors tend to cluster close to the triple negative group. They have a low to negative expression of estrogen receptor–related genes (ESR-1) and ERBB2 and related genes. Also, basal cytokeratins are inconsistently expressed. Additionally, the expression of proliferations markers is low in these tumors. This group of tumors, alternatively, seems to have an increased expression of genes related to the immune system, cell-cell communication, cell differentiation, cell migration, and angiogenesis. Decreased expression of genes related to cell-to-cell adhesion is also seen, such as the claudin group (3, 4, and 7) and E-cadherin. Morphologically, these tumors are

Table 1
Classification of breast carcinoma into intrinsic subtypes using immunohistochemistry

ER-Positive Tumors	ER-Negative Tumors
Luminal A • ER positive/Her-2/neu negative	ERBB2 • ER negative/Her-2/neu positive
Luminal B • ER positive/Her-2/neu negative/Ki-67 ≥ 14% • ER positive/Her-2/neu negative	Basal Phenotype • ER negative/Her-2/neu negative • Positive for HMW cytokeratins (eg, CK 5/6) and EGFR

heterogeneous, including metaplastic, medullary, and IDC-NOS. The overall prognosis and survival in these tumors are worse than luminal A and more akin to that of luminal B, ERBB2, and basal subtypes.[33]

Molecular Apocrine Subtype

Farmer and colleagues[34] identified another group of breast carcinomas, which include all ER-negative tumors (decreased expression of ESR1 gene), distinct from the basal-like group. These tumors overexpress ERRB2 genes and also show increased androgen receptor (AR) signaling. Other overexpressed genes include those related to metabolism (lipid synthesis). Correlation with apocrine morphology reveals a strong association between marked apocrine features and the AR+/ER- phenotype. Similar associations between apocrine morphology, ER negativity, and ERRB2 positivity have been reported,[35] suggesting an overlap between the ERRB2-enriched group and the molecular apocrine group. Coexpression of AR and Her-2/neu has also been reported by immunohistochemistry in a subset of high-grade invasive carcinomas with apocrine features.[36] One of the proposed hypotheses to explain this association suggests that ERRB2 overexpression stabilizes, modifies, and impacts AR function and expression.[37] Identifying genes that are overexpressed in molecular apocrine carcinomas, such as AR and HMGCR, will help design and use of novel treatment options tailored in these patients.[34]

Interferon-Related Group

More recently, an additional possible subtype has been described, namely, the interferon (IFN) group, which shows an increased proliferation of IFN-related genes including STAT1.[18] STAT1 is considered to regulate the overexpression of the IFN-related genes.[38] Overexpression of these genes has been associated with poor prognosis.

MOLECULAR CORRELATES OF HISTOLOGIC SUBTYPES

As per the World Health Organization's classification, 17 additional subtypes have been described based on specific morphologic features (**Table 2**). Tumors in each of these categories are defined by a constellation of morphologic features that are unique to that special type. Together, these tumors approximate 25% of all breast cancers.[2] These morphologic subtypes have, in the past, intrigued researchers; one of the questions, which arise from morphologic categorization of these tumors, is whether the morphology bears any independent prognostic and predictive significance. Studies have also documented a pathologist-dependent variability in diagnosing these subtypes.

Some morphologic variants have already been described to have characteristic clinical features. For example, tubular carcinomas are known to have an excellent prognosis with significantly longer disease-free and breast cancer–specific survival.[39] Similarly, cribriform carcinoma has also been reported to have a better disease-free survival[40] compared with grade 1 IDC-NOS. The morphologic variants within the triple-negative subtype also highlight the heterogeneity of this molecular subtype. To illustrate this, studies report the good prognosis of the adenoid cystic and medullary carcinoma compared with triple-negative IDC and, conversely, the relatively worse outcome of metaplastic carcinoma.[41] Also, the pathologic response achieved among the different variants, further underscore the importance of this knowledge.

Barring the usage of E-cadherin by immunohistochemistry, there are few identified and validated diagnostic markers that can be used appropriately to differentiate or

Table 2
Histologic subtypes and their molecular subtypes

Histologic Subtype	Molecular Subtype
Invasive lobular carcinoma	—
Classic variant	Luminal A
Pleomorphic variant	Luminal A ERBB2 enriched/molecular apocrine
Tubular carcinoma	Luminal A
Mucinous/neuroendocrine	Luminal A
Invasive papillary carcinoma	Luminal A
Micropapillary carcinoma	Luminal B/C ERRB2
Apocrine carcinoma	ERBB2 enriched/molecular apocrine Triple negative
Metaplastic carcinoma	Triple negative
Medullary carcinoma	Triple negative
Adenoid cystic carcinoma	Triple negative
Secretory carcinoma	Triple negative

Data from Weigelt B, Horlings HM, Kreike B, et al. Refinement of breast cancer classification by molecular characterization of histological special types. J Pathol 2008;216:141–50.

characterize these subtypes. This point brings forth another question: How different are these tumors at the molecular level and if these tumors bear any resemblance to the molecular subtypes thus far identified?

Weigelt and colleagues undertook a study, which included 113 cases of 11 pure histologic subtypes.[42] There were 1098 intrinsic genes analyzed, and hierarchical cluster analysis was performed. They were able to identify molecular subtypes for most histologic types studied. Mostly, each histologic type seemed to be relatively homogenous and correlated with one molecular subtype; however, some of the histologic variants seemed to be more heterogeneous and corresponded with multiple intrinsic subtypes.

Some of the selected and more commonly encountered special histologic subtypes, which are discussed in this article, include the following:

1. Invasive lobular carcinoma
2. Tubular carcinoma/cribriform
3. Invasive mucinous carcinoma/neuroendocrine carcinoma
4. Invasive papillary carcinoma
5. Invasive micropapillary carcinoma
6. Apocrine carcinoma
7. Metaplastic
8. Medullary
9. Secretory carcinoma
10. Adenoid cystic carcinoma

Invasive Lobular Carcinoma

Invasive lobular carcinoma accounts for 5% to 15% of all invasive carcinomas and is the most frequently encountered special type.[2] Discohesive cells characterize this histologic type morphologically, which may be singly dispersed or present as cords of cells in the stroma. Sometimes these cells may aggregate into small clusters (alveolar) and in a sheet-like pattern (solid). A definitive desmoplastic response is not seen associated with these neoplastic cells. In the classic variant, the nuclei are small (resembling a lymphocyte) and relatively uniform. The mitotic index is very low. Invasive lobular carcinoma seems to have distinct prognostic differences when compared with ductal carcinoma, with an early survival advantage.[43] These tumors are positive for estrogen and progesterone receptors and negative for Her-2/neu. Although they are predominantly of the luminal A subtype and fall into this cluster on unsupervised hierarchical clustering, they segregate independently of the luminal A ductal carcinoma, within this cluster.[44,45] In the recent past, another subtype of lobular carcinoma, the pleomorphic variant, is being increasingly described in the literature.[46,47] This variant is characterized with a high-grade cytology with apocrine features, pleomorphic nuclei, and exhibit a higher proliferation rate. Accurate identification of these tumors is of significant interest because these tumors seem to have a worse prognosis with a higher rate of recurrence when compared with high-grade ductal carcinoma and classic-type lobular carcinoma.[48,49] Most of these tumors are estrogen receptor positive and Her-2/neu negative, whereas a small subset of the pleomorphic variant may be estrogen receptor negative and Her-2/neu positive by immunohistochemistry. At the molecular level, these tumors predominantly prove to be of the luminal A subtype; rare cases are luminal B, ERBB2 enriched, and of the molecular apocrine subtype. Also, these tumors seem to be different at the molecular level from grade- and molecular subtype–matched IDC-NOS. Downregulated genes in ILC compared with IDC are the CDH1 gene and the genes associated with cell adhesion, cell cycle regulation, and cytoskeleton remodeling. Also downregulated differentially in lobular carcinoma is the TMSB10 gene, associated with cell growth and proliferation. Alternatively, genes that are upregulated are ESR2, and genes involved in lipid metabolism and PLEKHA7 gene which may play a role in invasion among others.[42,44] Most of these tumors reveal a 16q loss with a gain of 1q by CGH analysis. Other alterations, which differentiate them from ductal carcinoma, are 13q and 22q losses, which are seen more frequently in lobular carcinoma, whereas losses in 11q are more common in ductal carcinoma.[45]

Tubular Carcinoma/Cribriform Carcinoma

These tumors, composing approximately 4% of all breast carcinomas, are composed predominantly (>90%) of small, round to oval or angulated tubular structures with open lumina.[2] The cells lining the tubules are cuboidal, cytologically bland cells with a low mitotic index. Cribriform carcinomas, often associated with tubular carcinoma, are histologically characterized by a predominant cribriform growth pattern.

By immunohistochemistry, both of these histologic subtypes are positive for estrogen receptor and negative for Her-2/neu.

Tubular carcinomas seem to have a significantly better prognosis compared with low-grade IDC-NOS,[39] with a life expectancy approximating the general population. A similar good prognosis is also seen with cribriform carcinoma.[50]

At the molecular level, these tumors cluster with the luminal A subtype, indicating that they share similarities with these tumors at the genomic level.

Compared with grade- and molecular subtype–matched IDC-NOS, these tumors exhibit an upregulation of estrogen receptor-, transcription-, and apoptosis-related genes. Upregulation of the estrogen receptor signaling pathway seen in tubular carcinomas may explain the favorable prognosis that these tumors enjoy compared with grade-matched IDC-NOS.[42]

By CGH analysis, a loss of 16q has been documented in most of the tubular carcinoma cases studied (86%), with 52% cases showing a 2p loss and 48% cases showing a 9p loss. The most frequent (62%) chromosomal gains involve 11p and 13q.[51]

Mucinous and Neuroendocrine Carcinoma

These tumors are estimated at 2% of all invasive breast carcinomas.[2] Morphologically, they are composed of tumor cell nests and clusters accompanied by large pools of extracellular mucin making up more than 90% of the tumor. They are noted to have a lower incidence of lymph nodal involvement and a better overall survival when compared with IDC. These tumors have been divided into paucicellular and cellular groups (type A and B), respectively.[52] The type A tumors have a lower cell-to-mucus ratio, with 60% to 90% of the tumor being composed of mucus, whereas the hypercellular variant exhibits larger cell nests compared with the amount of mucin (30%–75% composed of mucin). These tumors are generally positive for estrogen receptor by immunohistochemistry and also for chromogranin and synaptophysin. The diagnosis of neuroendocrine carcinoma is made based on typical histologic features and when more than 50% of the cells were positive for neuroendocrine markers. On genomic analysis, these tumors correspond to the luminal A subtype.[42] Further hierarchical analysis concludes that within this group, type A mucinous tumors tend to form a separate cluster, whereas the type B and neuroendocrine tumors are intermixed. Overall, they seem to be a distinct group when compared with grade- and molecular subtype–matched IDC-NOS.[53] At the transcript level, mucinous A tumors show downregulation of extracellular matrix genes compared with grade- and subtype-matched IDC-NOS. Also downregulated are high-molecular cytokeratin genes and ERBB2, whereas estrogen receptor–regulated genes, BCL 2, luminal keratins, and genes of the FGF family seem to be upregulated in these tumors. In the mucinous B subtype, similar differences were seen as in mucinous A; in addition, the upregulation of the p53 and the Wnt/b-catenin signaling pathway is seen. Considerable overlap is seen between the luminal B and neuroendocrine tumors.[53] By CGH analysis, mucinous tumors showed gains of 1q and 16p and losses of 16q and 22q less frequently than grade- and ER-matched IDC-NOS. Also, the concurrent loss of 16q and gain of 1q, considered to be a characteristic feature of low-grade carcinomas, is not seen in pure mucinous tumors.[54]

Invasive Papillary Carcinoma

Papillary carcinomas of the breast in addition to the encapsulated papillary carcinoma may be invasive and of the solid papillary subtype. Neoplastic epithelial cells lining a fibrovascular core and the lack of a myoepithelial cell layer characterize papillary carcinoma. In the solid papillary variant, the neoplastic cells form solid, nodular nests surrounded by a fibrous capsule.

Most of these tumors are positive for estrogen receptor and negative for Her-2/neu (lumina A),[55,56] although lumina B, Her-2/neu overexpressing and triple-negative subtypes have been identified in smaller numbers.[56] Compared with matched cases of IDC-NOS, these tumors seem to have a better overall survival and disease-free survival. Additionally, the subtype status also shows a significant impact on survival.

These tumors do not cluster with grade- and ER-matched IDC-NOS on unsupervised hierarchical cluster analysis. Although the pattern of genomic aberrations are similar to that seen in IDC- NOS, the number of these changes are fewer and less complex.[55] Commonly seen are genomic alterations characteristic of ER-positive low-grade breast cancer, such as a loss of 16q and gains in 16p and 1q. The most commonly encountered amplification is CCND1 gene amplification, located on 11q13, seen in about one-tenth of the cases.[55] Also, PIK3CA mutations were more frequently seen in papillary carcinoma cases compared with grade- and ER-matched IDC-NOS.

Finally, the 3 variants of papillary carcinoma, encapsulated papillary carcinoma, solid papillary carcinoma, and invasive papillary carcinoma, do not cluster independently of each other on unsupervised hierarchical clustering and may represent variations of the same pathologic entity.

Invasive Micropapillary Carcinoma

Pure or predominantly micropapillary carcinomas constitute less the 2% of all breast cancer cases.[2] Morphologically, these tumors have a very distinctive architectural pattern and are composed of nests of tumor cells with reversed polarity present within the lacunar spaces. An abluminal staining pattern with Epithelial Membrane Antigen (EMA) is useful in demonstrating the reverse polarity of the cells. Micropapillary carcinomas are variably positive for estrogen receptor and Her-2/neu. They tend to have a higher rate of lymph node metastasis compared with IDC-NOS. Also, a worse prognosis has been attributed to these tumors.[57] These tumors tend to be predominantly of the luminal subtype with a smaller subset being of the Her-2 phenotype.[58] Also associated with these tumors is a high proliferation index, indicating that they belong to the luminal B subtype rather than luminal A.[58] Rare triple-negative cases have also been reported.[59]

Complex genomic alterations have been identified in this variant using CGH technology. The most frequent alteration seen is the loss of 8p. Other chromosomal alterations include the loss of 1p, 17p, and 16q. Also, approximately two-thirds of these cases showed evidence of a 6p gain and a 6q loss.[58] Gains are seen in 16p, 1q, 17q, 13q, 8p, and 1p. Recurrent amplifications were reported in 4p, 8p, 8q, 11q, 17q, and 20q. Amplification of 8q has been significantly associated with micropapillary carcinoma,[58,60] compared with ductal carcinomas, and these amplified regions include the MYC gene. Amplification of the MYC gene has been reported in one-third of the cases; this has been linked to proliferation, metastasis, and aggressive behavior.[58]

Compared with grade- and ER-matched IDC-NOS, micropapillary carcinomas tend to be genetically more complex more frequently and seem to be a distinct entity.

Apocrine Carcinoma

These carcinomas are defined as carcinomas with more than 90% of the tumor exhibiting apocrine differentiation, which includes eosinophilic cytoplasm, round nuclei, and prominent nucleoli. In some cases, the cytoplasm may be finely vacuolated. They are relatively rare and constitute 0.3% to 4.0% of all breast carcinomas.[2] These tumors are frequently positive for GCDFP 15 by immunohistochemistry. Most of these tumors tend to be estrogen receptor negative, AR positive, and Her-2/neu negative, whereas the rest are estrogen receptor negative and AR and Her-2/neu receptor positive.[61,62] In addition, p53 overexpression is significantly associated with the triple-negative apocrine group.[62]

In addition to the morphologic features, this subtype has also been shown to exist as a distinct entity at the molecular level by gene expression profiling.[34]

Clinically, studies have shown that these tumors have a significantly worse overall disease-free survival compared with IDC. Also, reporting the AR status of these patients may be important because they could potentially benefit from targeted therapy.

Metaplastic Carcinoma

These carcinomas are a morphologically heterogeneous group of tumors, which constitute less than 1% of all breast carcinomas.[2] They are composed of an admixture of adenocarcinoma with a spindle cell, squamous, or mesenchymal component. In some cases, the spindle cell and squamous cell components may be pure, lacking an admixed adenocarcinoma component. These tumors are hormone receptor and Her-2/neu negative. Clinically, they are aggressive tumors and seem to be more chemoresistant when compared with other triple-negative tumors.[63] With gene expression profiling and unsupervised hierarchical clustering, metaplastic carcinomas cluster with and are intermixed with basal-like ductal carcinoma. At the transcriptional level, differential expression of genes between the 2 groups is seen, clinically relevant among these being the downregulation of the PTEN and TOP2A genes in metaplastic carcinoma, which are targets for anthracyclines and, therefore, may explain chemoresistance to these agents.[42,64] Also, another study looking at the genome-wide analysis of different components of these tumors reported genetic heterogeneity, which corresponds with the morphologic variations present.[65] A high proportion of alterations related to the PI3K/AKT pathway have been identified in these tumors. Additionally, these tumors exhibit a high-level genomic instability based on the proportion of genetic alterations present. Gains in 1p, 11q, 12q, 14q, 22q, and 19p and an increased loss of 1q, 2p, 3q, and 8q are seen. A gain in 1q and a loss of 16q, alterations generally present in low-grade tumors, are not seen.[63] Although they are triple-negative and they seem to cluster adjacent to the basal tumors by hierarchical clustering, at the transcriptional level, metaplastic tumors seem to be a distinct subset from the basal-like tumors.

Medullary Carcinoma

Tumors included in this histologic subtype have well-defined pushing borders, high-grade cytology with pleomorphic and vesicular nuclei, and numerous mitoses and syncytial growth patterns. Tubule formation and in situ components are not seen. A prominent tumoral lymphocytic infiltrate is present. These carcinomas compose 1% to 7% of all breast carcinomas, and this variation depends on the criteria used for diagnosis.[2] These tumors are predominantly estrogen receptor negative; however, cases that are estrogen positive have been described.[66] Although the rate of progesterone receptor positivity is low, this seems to confer some survival benefit to these patients. According to some studies, these tumors reportedly have a better overall survival when compared with IDC-NOS.[66–68] However, lymph node metastasis, size of the tumor, and distant metastasis seem to decrease the overall survival in these patients.[66,69,70] At the molecular level, these tumors cluster with the basal tumors, illustrating a lack of expression of the ESR and Her-2/neu genes.[42,71] However, some differences have been reported. Compared with basal-like tumors, medullary carcinomas showed increased expression of immune response genes, including T cell–associated genes, STAT 1, and IFN-regulating genes, such as IRF1, IRF7, IRF2, IRF4, and IRF 8. Also seen is an overexpression of apoptosis-related genes, such as tumor necrosis factor (TNF) receptor genes, TNF ligand superfamilies, and TNFα-induced proteins. Underexpressed genes included those related to the maintenance of the cytoskeleton, including actins, myosin, and tropomyosin. Compared with basal-like cancers, there is a loss of expression of myoepithelial-related genes.[71] Medullary breast carcinomas show gains in chromosomes 1q, 8p, 10p, and 12p, which have not been reported in basal like carcinoma (BLC).[72] Medullary features are also seen frequently in BRCA1 mutation–related tumors, approximating 11%.

Although these tumors are triple negative and seem similar to basal-like cancers at a glance, there are genetic/molecular differences between them, which may explain the good prognosis associated with them.

Secretory Carcinoma

These tumors are identified by the presence of eosinophilic secretions present in intracellular vacuoles and spaces. They are extremely rare tumors and compose less than 0.15% of all breast cancers. Originally described in young patients, they were termed "juvenile carcinomas"[73]; however, with subsequent identification in adult patients, the terminology was changed to *secretory carcinoma* based on the very characteristic morphology of these tumors.[74]

These tumors are typically slow growing, with rare instances of lymph node metastasis if any. Most of these cases are triple negative, although rare cases with hormone receptor positivity have been reported. In addition, reports of these tumors document them to be positive for basal cytokeratins, C-KIT, and EGFR.[75,76] The occurrence of these rather indolent tumors as triple negative highlights the increasingly recognized heterogeneity of this group of tumors. Chromosomal translocation (t12; 15) resulting in the fusion of the ETSV6 and NTRK3 genes, although not consistently present, is considered characteristic for secretory carcinoma.[76,77]

Adenoid Cystic Carcinoma

Adenoid cystic carcinoma of the breast is an extremely rare subtype and composes about 0.1% of all breast carcinomas.[2] Histologically, they mimic the adenoid cystic tumor of the salivary gland, with the tumor cells resembling epithelial-myoepithelial cells. These cells are arranged in cords, cribriform, and solid nests and are associated with eosinophilic hyaline basement membrane–like material and mucoid material. Mitoses are rare. The basal cells express basal cytokeratins, p63, actin, calponin, and S 100, whereas the luminal cells express luminal cytokeratin, EMA, carcinoembryonic antigen (CEA), and C-KIT. Typically, these tumors are negative for estrogen receptors and Her-2/neu by immunohistochemistry.

Compared with IDC-NOS of a similar grade, these tumors are reported to have a significantly better prognosis and overall survival. Axillary lymph node metastasis is rarely seen in these tumors; therefore, axillary node dissection is not considered essential.

These tumors cluster with the basal subtype by gene expression profiling. However, there seems to be downregulation of genes involved in migration, proliferation, and invasion, possibly underlying the good prognosis in these patients.[42] The genomic alterations seem to differ from grade-matched IDC cases. A repeated genetic abnormality that has bee detected in adenoid cystic carcinoma of both the breast and head and neck is the fusion of MYB and NFIB transcription factors, which results from t (6;9). This abnormality has not been detected in grade-matched triple-negative breast carcinoma cases.[78–80]

DUCTAL CARCINOMA IN SITU

Since the institution of mammographic screening for breast cancer, the diagnosis of ductal carcinoma in situ (DCIS) has increased many fold in the recent decades, composing approximately 20% of all breast carcinoma diagnoses. Although DCIS is a nonobligate precursor of invasive carcinoma, a diagnosis of DCIS increases the risk of subsequent invasive carcinoma 8 to 10 times. Without treatment, approximately half of the cases of DCIS will transform to invasive carcinoma.[81] Traditionally, DCIS is classified by an architectural growth pattern, nuclear grade, and the presence or absence of necrosis. A nuclear grade is considered to have prognostic significance, with DCIS of a high nuclear grade having the highest recurrence rate (reviewed in Ref.[82]).

The biologic markers estrogen and progesterone receptors are positive in approximately half to three-fourths of the in situ lesions, and these hormone receptor–positive cases are associated with a low nuclear grade and noncomedo carcinomas.[83–85] Her-2/neu expression has been reported in 30% to 55% of DCIS and has been associated with high nuclear grade. Provenzano and colleagues[86] reported that a negative status of hormone receptors and a positive Her2 status were independent prognostic markers. Additionally, p53 protein expression has been reported in high-grade DCIS.[87]

Studies that have analyzed gene expression at the RNA level have identified heterogeneity at the molecular level in these precursor lesions. Using 392 genes to identify the intrinsic subtypes, luminal, basal, and ERBB2 subtypes were identified within the in situ lesions, which underscores the hypothesis that molecular abnormalities and alterations are acquired early in the neoplastic process.[88]

IN SITU TO INVASIVE CARCINOMA: MOLECULAR PATHWAYS?

Two models of progression of DCIS to invasive cancer have been hypothesized. The first model is known as the *theory of linear progression*, which purports that low-grade DCIS progresses to high-grade DCIS and then transforms to invasive cancer. The second theory, also known as the *theory of parallel disease* proposes that low-grade DCIS transforms into low-grade invasive carcinoma and high-grade DCIS progresses to high-grade invasive carcinoma (reviewed in Ref.[89]). A study by Gupta and colleagues[90] has shown that the grade of DCIS and concurrent invasive carcinoma are correlated, and this is also correlated with the outcome. A more recent study by Wallis and colleagues[91] concluded that high-grade DCIS tends to recur earlier than low-grade DCIS. Also, in their study cohort of patients with low-grade DCIS, the investigators did not identify any high-grade recurrences, metastases, or deaths. Molecular studies also support this theory to be more likely involved in breast cancer progression. One such finding in support of this particular theory is that the loss of chromosome 16q is seen more frequently in low-grade DCIS, whereas allelic imbalances of 13q, 17q, and 20q are more common in high-grade DCIS. These changes are recapitulated or maintained in concurrent invasive lesions.[92] Although the aforementioned studies support the theory of parallel disease, they also imply that these 2 pathways may not be mutually exclusive. This point is also exemplified in another study whereby the investigators identified a subset of low-grade DCIS that eventually developed high-grade DCIS.[93]

The tipping point in the progression of in situ carcinoma to invasive carcinoma is characterized by the breach of the basement membrane and invasion of the stroma. Studies have illustrated differences at the molecular level, when comparing stroma surrounding DCIS to stroma around invasive disease.[94,95] Looking at cases of pure DCIS versus cases associated with invasive disease, upregulation of genes related to Epithelial-Mesenchymal Transition (EMT) and myoepithelial cells have been reported in the epithelial compartment of the latter when compared with epithelium of pure DCIS.[96] In contrast, the epithelial component of DCIS associated with invasive disease is very similar to the invasive component.[94,95] This point brings forth the implication that pure DCIS might be a distinct disease compared with DCIS associated with invasion, at the molecular level.

Although the exact pathway of progression of DCIS is still under investigation and remains debatable, it seems that genetic/transcriptional changes in both epithelial and stromal compartments are essential to this process.

SUMMARY

The most significant contribution of molecular subtyping of breast carcinomas has been the identification of estrogen-positive and estrogen-negative tumor subtypes. These subtypes are 2 distinct entities with differing prognoses and requiring a different therapy. Also, molecular and genetic analyses can provide prognostic information; however, a thorough histopathologic evaluation with the evaluation of the predictive biomarkers (Estrogen and Progesterone Receptors and Her-2/neu) is able to provide similar information. Knowledge of genetic alterations in these tumors will help us identify novel therapeutic targets, which might have a significant impact on prognosis. Finally, understanding the progression pathways involved in the transition of in situ carcinoma to invasive carcinoma might lead to efficient risk stratification in these patients.

REFERENCES

1. Siegel R, Naishadham D, Jemal A. Cancer statistics, 2013. CA Cancer J Clin 2013;63:11–30.
2. Tavassoli FA, Devilee P, editors. World Health Organization classification of tumor. Pathology and genetics of tumors of the breast and female genital organs. Lyon (France): IARC Press; 2003. p. 13–59.
3. O'Brien KM, Cole SR, Tse CK, et al. Intrinsic breast tumor subtypes, race, and long-term survival in the Carolina Breast Cancer Study. Clin Cancer Res 2010; 16:6100–10.
4. Patani N, Martin LA, Dowsett M. Biomarkers for the clinical management of breast cancer: international perspective. Int J Cancer 2013;133(1):1–13.
5. Hammond ME. ASCO-CAP guidelines for breast predictive factor testing: an update. Appl Immunohistochem Mol Morphol 2011;19:499–500.
6. Perou CM, Sorlie T, Eisen MB, et al. Molecular portraits of human breast tumours. Nature 2000;406:747–52.
7. Sorlie T, Perou CM, Tibshirani R, et al. Gene expression patterns of breast carcinomas distinguish tumor subclasses with clinical implications. Proc Natl Acad Sci U S A 2001;98:10869–74.
8. Sotiriou C, Neo SY, McShane LM, et al. Breast cancer classification and prognosis based on gene expression profiles from a population-based study. Proc Natl Acad Sci U S A 2003;100:10393–8.
9. Prat A, Cheang MC, Martin M, et al. Prognostic significance of progesterone receptor-positive tumor cells within immunohistochemically defined luminal A breast cancer. J Clin Oncol 2013;31:203–9.
10. Park S, Koo JS, Kim MS, et al. Characteristics and outcomes according to molecular subtypes of breast cancer as classified by a panel of four biomarkers using immunohistochemistry. Breast 2012;21:50–7.
11. Voduc KD, Cheang MC, Tyldesley S, et al. Breast cancer subtypes and the risk of local and regional relapse. J Clin Oncol 2010;28:1684–91.
12. Goldhirsch A, Wood WC, Coates AS, et al. Strategies for subtypes–dealing with the diversity of breast cancer: highlights of the St. Gallen International Expert Consensus on the Primary Therapy of Early Breast Cancer 2011. Ann Oncol 2011;22:1736–47.
13. Kim HS, Park I, Cho HJ, et al. Analysis of the potent prognostic factors in luminal-type breast cancer. J Breast Cancer 2012;15:401–6.
14. Cheang MC, Chia SK, Voduc D, et al. Ki67 index, HER2 status, and prognosis of patients with luminal B breast cancer. J Natl Cancer Inst 2009;101:736–50.

15. Wirapati P, Sotiriou C, Kunkel S, et al. Meta-analysis of gene expression profiles in breast cancer: toward a unified understanding of breast cancer subtyping and prognosis signatures. Breast Cancer Res 2008;10:R65.

16. Guiu S, Michiels S, Andre F, et al. Molecular subclasses of breast cancer: how do we define them? the IMPAKT 2012 Working Group Statement. Ann Oncol 2012;23:2997–3006.

17. Ono M, Tsuda H, Yunokawa M, et al. Prognostic impact of Ki-67 labeling indices with 3 different cutoff values, histological grade, and nuclear grade in hormone-receptor-positive, HER2-negative, node-negative invasive breast cancers. Breast Cancer 2013. [Epub ahead of print].

18. Hu Z, Fan C, Oh DS, et al. The molecular portraits of breast tumors are conserved across microarray platforms. BMC Genomics 2006;7:96.

19. Natrajan R, Weigelt B, Mackay A, et al. An integrative genomic and transcrip-tomic analysis reveals molecular pathways and networks regulated by copy number aberrations in basal-like, HER2 and luminal cancers. Breast Cancer Res Treat 2010;121:575–89.

20. Wiechmann L, Sampson M, Stempel M, et al. Presenting features of breast can-cer differ by molecular subtype. Ann Surg Oncol 2009;16:2705–10.

21. Dowsett M, Procter M, McCaskill-Stevens W, et al. Disease-free survival accord-ing to degree of HER2 amplification for patients treated with adjuvant chemo-therapy with or without 1 year of trastuzumab: the HERA Trial. J Clin Oncol 2009;27:2962–9.

22. Smith I, Procter M, Gelber RD, et al, HERA study team. 2-year follow-up of tras-tuzumab after adjuvant chemotherapy in HER2-positive breast cancer: a rand-omised controlled trial. Lancet 2007;369:29–36.

23. Gennari A, Sormani MP, Pronzato P, et al. HER2 status and efficacy of adjuvant anthracyclines in early breast cancer: a pooled analysis of randomized trials. J Natl Cancer Inst 2008;100:14–20.

24. Hayes DF, Thor AD, Dressler LG, et al, Cancer and Leukemia Group B (CALGB) Investigators. HER2 and response to paclitaxel in node-positive breast cancer. N Engl J Med 2007;357:1496–506.

25. Pritchard KI, Messersmith H, Elavathil L, et al. HER-2 and topoisomerase II as predictors of response to chemotherapy. J Clin Oncol 2008;26:736–44.

26. Goldstein NS, Decker D, Severson D, et al. Molecular classification system iden-tifies invasive breast carcinoma patients who are most likely and those who are least likely to achieve a complete pathologic response after neoadjuvant chemotherapy. Cancer 2007;110:1687–96.

27. Nguyen PL, Taghian AG, Katz MS, et al. Breast cancer subtype approximated by estrogen receptor, progesterone receptor, and HER-2 is associated with local and distant recurrence after breast-conserving therapy. J Clin Oncol 2008;26:2373–8.

28. Kennecke H, Yerushalmi R, Woods R, et al. Metastatic behavior of breast cancer subtypes. J Clin Oncol 2010;28:3271–7.

29. Smid M, Wang Y, Zhang Y, et al. Subtypes of breast cancer show preferential site of relapse. Cancer Res 2008;68:3108–14.

30. Livasy CA, Karaca G, Nanda R, et al. Phenotypic evaluation of the basal-like subtype of invasive breast carcinoma. Mod Pathol 2006;19:264–71.

31. Bosch A, Eroles P, Zaragoza R, et al. Triple-negative breast cancer: molecular features, pathogenesis, treatment and current lines of research. Cancer Treat Rev 2010;36:206–15.

32. Carey LA, Perou CM, Livasy CA, et al. Race, breast cancer subtypes, and sur-vival in the Carolina Breast Cancer Study. JAMA 2006;295:2492–502.

33. Prat A, Parker JS, Karginova O, et al. Phenotypic and molecular characterization of the claudin-low intrinsic subtype of breast cancer. Breast Cancer Res 2010; 12:R68.

34. Farmer P, Bonnefoi H, Becette V, et al. Identification of molecular apocrine breast tumours by microarray analysis. Oncogene 2005;24:4660–71.

35. Bhargava R, Striebel J, Beriwal S, et al. Prevalence, morphologic features and proliferation indices of breast carcinoma molecular classes using immunohisto-chemical surrogate markers. Int J Clin Exp Pathol 2009;2:444–55.

36. Moinfar F, Okcu M, Tsybrovskyy O, et al. Androgen receptors frequently are expressed in breast carcinomas: potential relevance to new therapeutic strategies. Cancer 2003;98:703–11.

37. Mellinghoff IK, Vivanco I, Kwon A, et al. HER2/neu kinase-dependent modulation of androgen receptor function through effects on DNA binding and stability. Cancer Cell 2004;6:517–27.

38. Bromberg JF, Horvath CM, Wen Z, et al. Transcriptionally active Stat1 is required for the antiproliferative effects of both interferon alpha and interferon gamma. Proc Natl Acad Sci U S A 1996;93:7673–8.

39. Rakha EA, Lee AH, Evans AJ, et al. Tubular carcinoma of the breast: further evidence to support its excellent prognosis. J Clin Oncol 2010;28:99–104.

40. Colleoni M, Rotmensz N, Maisonneuve P, et al. Outcome of special types of luminal breast cancer. Ann Oncol 2012;23:1428–36.

41. Montagna E, Maisonneuve P, Rotmensz N, et al. Heterogeneity of triple-negative breast cancer: histologic subtyping to inform the outcome. Clin Breast Cancer 2013;13:31–9.

42. Weigelt B, Horlings HM, Kreike B, et al. Refinement of breast cancer classification by molecular characterization of histological special types. J Pathol 2008; 216:141–50.

43. Iorfida M, Maiorano E, Orvieto E, et al. Invasive lobular breast cancer: subtypes and outcome. Breast Cancer Res Treat 2012;133:713–23.

44. Castellana B, Escuin D, Perez-Olabarria M, et al. Genetic up-regulation and overexpression of PLEKHA7 differentiates invasive lobular carcinomas from invasive ductal carcinomas. Hum Pathol 2012;43:1902–9.

45. Gruel N, Lucchesi C, Raynal V, et al. Lobular invasive carcinoma of the breast is a molecular entity distinct from luminal invasive ductal carcinoma. Eur J Cancer 2010;46:2399–407.

46. Eusebi V, Magalhaes F, Azzopardi AG. Pleomorphic lobular carcinoma of the breast: an aggressive tumor showing apocrine differentiation. Hum Pathol 1992;23:655–62.

47. Middleton LP, Palacios DM, Bryant BR, et al. Pleomorphic lobular carcinoma: morphology, immunocytochemistry and molecular analysis. Am J Surg Pathol 2000;24:1650–6.

48. Monhollen L, Morrison C, Ademuyiwa FO, et al. Pleomorphic lobular carcinoma: a distinctive clinical and molecular breast cancer type. Histopathology 2012;61: 365–77.

49. Buchanan CL, Flynn LW, Murray MP, et al. Is pleomorphic lobular carcinoma really a distinct clinical entity? J Surg Oncol 2008;98:314–7.

50. Venable JG, Schwartz AM, Silverberg SG. Infiltrating cribriform carcinoma of the breast: a distinctive clinicopathologic entity. Hum Pathol 1990;21:333–8.

51. Riener MO, Nikolopoulos E, Herr A, et al. Microarray comparative genomic hybridization analysis of tubular breast carcinoma shows recurrent loss of the CDH13 locus on 16q. Hum Pathol 2008;39:1621–9.

52. Capella C, Eusebi V, Mann B, et al. Endocrine differentiation in mucoid carcinoma of the breast. Histopathology 1980;4:613–30.
53. Weigelt B, Geyer FC, Horlings HM, et al. Mucinous and neuroendocrine breast carcinomas are transcriptionally distinct from invasive ductal carcinomas of no special type. Mod Pathol 2009;22:1401–14.
54. Lacroix-Triki M, Suarez PH, MacKay A, et al. Mucinous carcinoma of the breast is genomically distinct from invasive ductal carcinomas of no special type. J Pathol 2010;222:282–98.
55. Duprez R, Wilkerson PM, Lacroix-Triki M, et al. Immunophenotypic and genomic characterization of papillary carcinomas of the breast. J Pathol 2012;226: 427–41.
56. Liu ZY, Liu N, Wang YH, et al. Clinicopathologic characteristics and molecular subtypes of invasive papillary carcinoma of the breast: a large case study. J Cancer Res Clin Oncol 2013;139:77–84.
57. Chen L, Fan Y, Lang RG, et al. Breast carcinoma with micropapillary features: clinicopathologic study and long-term follow-up of 100 cases. Int J Surg Pathol 2008;16:155–63.
58. Marchio C, Iravani M, Natrajan R, et al. Genomic and immunophenotypical characterization of pure micropapillary carcinomas of the breast. J Pathol 2008;215: 398–410.
59. Yamaguchi R, Tanaka M, Kondo K, et al. Characteristic morphology of invasive micropapillary carcinoma of the breast: an immunohistochemical analysis. Jpn J Clin Oncol 2010;40:781–7.
60. Thor AD, Eng C, Devries S, et al. Invasive micropapillary carcinoma of the breast is associated with chromosome 8 abnormalities detected by comparative genomic hybridization. Hum Pathol 2002;33:628–31.
61. Dellapasqua S, Maisonneuve P, Viale G, et al. Immunohistochemically defined subtypes and outcome of apocrine breast cancer. Clin Breast Cancer 2013; 13:95–102.
62. Tsutsumi Y. Apocrine carcinoma as triple-negative breast cancer: novel definition of apocrine-type carcinoma as estrogen/progesterone receptor-negative and androgen receptor-positive invasive ductal carcinoma. Jpn J Clin Oncol 2012;42:375–86.
63. Hennessy BT, Gonzalez-Angulo AM, Stemke-Hale K, et al. Characterization of a naturally occurring breast cancer subset enriched in epithelial-to-mesenchymal transition and stem cell characteristics. Cancer Res 2009;69: 4116–24.
64. Weigelt B, Kreike B, Reis-Filho JS. Metaplastic breast carcinomas are basal-like breast cancers: a genomic profiling analysis. Breast Cancer Res Treat 2009; 117:273–80.
65. Geyer FC, Weigelt B, Natrajan R, et al. Molecular analysis reveals a genetic basis for the phenotypic diversity of metaplastic breast carcinomas. J Pathol 2010; 220:562–73.
66. Martinez SR, Beal SH, Canter RJ, et al. Medullary carcinoma of the breast: a population-based perspective. Med Oncol 2011;28:738–44.
67. Li CI. Risk of mortality by histologic type of breast cancer in the United States. Hormones & cancer 2010;1:156–65.
68. Vu-Nishino H, Tavassoli FA, Ahrens WA, et al. Clinicopathologic features and long-term outcome of patients with medullary breast carcinoma managed with breast-conserving therapy (BCT). International Journal of Radiation Oncology, Biology, Physics 2005;62:1040–7.

69. Reinfuss M, Stelmach A, Mitus J, et al. Typical medullary carcinoma of the breast: a clinical and pathological analysis of 52 cases. Journal of Surgical Oncology 1995;60:89–94.

70. Ridolfi RL, Rosen PP, Port A, et al. Medullary carcinoma of the breast: a clinicopathologic study with 10 year follow-up. Cancer 1977;40:1365–85.

71. Bertucci F, Finetti P, Cervera N, et al. Gene expression profiling shows medullary breast cancer is a subgroup of basal breast cancers. Cancer Res 2006;66: 4636–44.

72. Vincent-Salomon A, Gruel N, Lucchesi C, et al. Identification of typical medullary breast carcinoma as a genomic sub-group of basal-like carcinomas, a heterogeneous new molecular entity. Breast Cancer Res 2007;9:R24.

73. McDivitt RW, Stewart FW. Breast carcinoma in children. JAMA 1966;195:388–90.

74. Oberman HA. Secretory carcinoma of the breast in adults. Am J Surg Pathol 1980;4:465–70.

75. Lae M, Freneaux P, Sastre-Garau X, et al. Secretory breast carcinomas with ETV6-NTRK3 fusion gene belong to the basal-like carcinoma spectrum. Mod Pathol 2009;22:291–8.

76. Lambros MB, Tan DS, Jones RL, et al. Genomic profile of a secretory breast cancer with an ETV6-NTRK3 duplication. J Clin Pathol 2009;62:604–12.

77. Vasudev P, Onuma K. Secretory breast carcinoma: unique, triple-negative carcinoma with a favorable prognosis and characteristic molecular expression. Arch Pathol Lab Med 2011;135:1606–10.

78. Brill LB 2nd, Kanner WA, Fehr A, et al. Analysis of MYB expression and MYB-NFIB gene fusions in adenoid cystic carcinoma and other salivary neoplasms. Mod Pathol 2011;24:1169–76.

79. Wetterskog D, Lopez-Garcia MA, Lambros MB, et al. Adenoid cystic carcinomas constitute a genomically distinct subgroup of triple-negative and basal-like breast cancers. J Pathol 2012;226:84–96.

80. Persson M, Andren Y, Mark J, et al. Recurrent fusion of MYB and NFIB transcription factor genes in carcinomas of the breast and head and neck. Proc Natl Acad Sci U S A 2009;106:18740–4.

81. Collins LC, Tamimi RM, Baer HJ, et al. Outcome of patients with ductal carcinoma in situ untreated after diagnostic biopsy: results from the Nurses' Health Study. Cancer 2005;103:1778–84.

82. Tsikitis VL, Chung MA. Biology of ductal carcinoma in situ classification based on biologic potential. Am J Clin Oncol 2006;29:305–10.

83. Chaudhuri B, Crist KA, Mucci S, et al. Distribution of estrogen receptor in ductal carcinoma in situ of the breast. Surgery 1993;113:134–7.

84. Barnes R, Masood S. Potential value of hormone receptor assay in carcinoma in situ of breast. Am J Clin Pathol 1990;94:533–7.

85. Karayiannakis AJ, Bastounis EA, Chatzigianni EB, et al. Immunohistochemical detection of oestrogen receptors in ductal carcinoma in situ of the breast. Eur J Surg Oncol 1996;22:578–82.

86. Provenzano E, Hopper JL, Giles GG, et al. Biological markers that predict clinical recurrence in ductal carcinoma in situ of the breast. Eur J Cancer 2003;39: 622–30.

87. Poller DN, Roberts EC, Bell JA, et al. p53 protein expression in mammary ductal carcinoma in situ: relationship to immunohistochemical expression of estrogen receptor and c-erbB-2 protein. Hum Pathol 1993;24:463–8.

88. Allred DC, Wu Y, Mao S, et al. Ductal carcinoma in situ and the emergence of diversity during breast cancer evolution. Clin Cancer Res 2008;14:370–8.

89. Wiechmann L, Kuerer HM. The molecular journey from ductal carcinoma in situ to invasive breast cancer. Cancer 2008;112:2130–42.

90. Gupta SK, Douglas-Jones AG, Fenn N, et al. The clinical behavior of breast carcinoma is probably determined at the preinvasive stage (ductal carcinoma in situ). Cancer 1997;80:1740–5.

91. Wallis MG, Clements K, Kearins O, et al. The effect of DCIS grade on rate, type and time to recurrence after 15 years of follow-up of screen-detected DCIS. Br J Cancer 2012;106:1611–7.

92. Reis-Filho JS, Lakhani SR. The diagnosis and management of pre-invasive breast disease: genetic alterations in pre-invasive lesions. Breast Cancer Res 2003;5:313–9.

93. King TA, Sakr RA, Muhsen S, et al. Is there a low-grade precursor pathway in breast cancer? Ann Surg Oncol 2012;19:1115–21.

94. Allinen M, Beroukhim R, Cai L, et al. Molecular characterization of the tumor microenvironment in breast cancer. Cancer Cell 2004;6:17–32.

95. Ma XJ, Salunga R, Tuggle JT, et al. Gene expression profiles of human breast cancer progression. Proc Natl Acad Sci U S A 2003;100:5974–9.

96. Knudsen ES, Ertel A, Davicioni E, et al. Progression of ductal carcinoma in situ to invasive breast cancer is associated with gene expression programs of EMT and myoepithelia. Breast Cancer Res Treat 2012;133:1009–24.

Gynecologic Cancers
Molecular Updates

Quratulain Ahmed, MD, Baraa Alosh, MD,
Sudeshna Bandyopadhyay, MD*, Rouba Ali-Fehmi, MD

KEYWORDS

- Molecular pathogenesis • Ovarian carcinoma • Uterine carcinoma
- Endometrial carcinoma

KEY POINTS

- Understanding the molecular basis of endometrial carcinoma helps to provide an explanation for the prognosis of these tumors.
- This understanding opens up avenues for research into novel therapies that may prove beneficial.

MOLECULAR PATHOGENESIS OF EPITHELIAL OVARIAN CANCER

Globally, ovarian cancer is the sixth most common cancer in women and ranks seventh among the most lethal cancers. The estimated number of new cases yearly is about 204,000 and there are 125,000 deaths annually.[1] In the United States, there are 22,240 new cases and 14,030 deaths from ovarian cancer annually.[2]

The new molecular studies led to a division of ovarian cancer into 2 types based on clinical, pathologic, and genetic features. A dualistic model of ovarian carcinogenesis has been proposed. Type I tumors include low-grade endometrioid, low-grade serous, clear cell, mucinous, and Brenner tumors. The behavior of these tumors is not aggressive and they are usually confined to the ovaries (FIGO stage I). The indolent progression of type I tumors reflects their relative genetic stability and they have multiple types of somatic mutations such as *KRAS*, *PTEN*, *BRAF*, *CTNNB*, *PIK3CA*, *PPP2R1A*, *ARID1A*, and rarely *TP53*.[3,4] Type II tumors include high-grade serous carcinoma, high-grade endometrioid, malignant mixed müllerian tumor, and undifferentiated carcinoma. The behavior of these tumors is more aggressive in comparison with type I tumors and they invade rapidly (FIGO stage II–IV). The genetic characteristics are highly unstable and *TP53* mutations are present in more than 95% of cases.[5] The mutations that exist in type I are rarely found in type II; *P53* mutations are mostly restricted to type II.[6]

Department of Pathology, Wayne State University, 540, E Canfield, Detroit, MI 48201, USA
* Corresponding author.
E-mail address: sbandyop@dmc.org

Clin Lab Med 33 (2013) 911–925
http://dx.doi.org/10.1016/j.cll.2013.09.001
0272-2712/13/$ – see front matter © 2013 Elsevier Inc. All rights reserved.
labmed.theclinics.com

Type I Tumors

Low-grade serous carcinoma

Low-grade serous carcinoma (LGSC) represents a minority of ovarian serous carcinomas.[7] The morphologic and genetic evidence support the notion that cystadenomas/adenofibromas are precursors of LGSC. In this model, serous cystadenoma progresses to an atypical proliferative serous tumor, noninvasive micropapillary serous carcinoma, and finally to invasive LGSC.[8]

It is widely accepted that high-grade serous carcinoma (HGSC) and LGSC are different type of tumors and have distinctive characteristics. LGSCs have a strong association with serous borderline tumors and express *KRAS* and *BRAF* mutations and do not express *TP53* mutations, which have a strong expression in HGSCs.[9] Epidemiology studies have showed the differences in survival, age, annual incidence, and other parameters between LGSC and HGSC.[7] These data support the distinct identity of LGSC in comparison with HGSC.

Clear cell carcinoma

The presentation of clear cell carcinoma of the ovary (**Fig. 1**D) is characterized by a large adnexal mass, FIGO stage I, and highly malignant behavior. Some studies suggest clear cell fibroadenoma can be a clonal precursor of clear cell carcinoma. This evidence for this association was provided by the identical loss of heterozygosity pattern in both clear cell fibroadenoma and clear cell carcinoma.[10] In addition, there is a well-known association between clear cell carcinoma and endometriosis.[11] Retrograde menstruation has been suggested as a mechanism of endometriotic implants; however, the origin of endometriosis has not been firmly established. Based on many genetic and molecular studies, the most common genetic abnormality is an inactivating mutation of *ARID1A* in 50% of tumors,[4] an activating mutation of *PIK3CA*

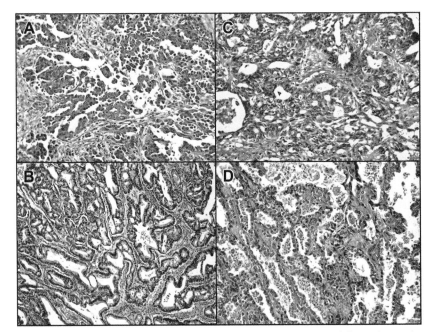

Fig. 1. (*A*) Ovarian serous carcinoma. (*B*) Ovarian mucinous carcinoma. (*C*) Ovarian endometrioid carcinoma. (*D*) Ovarian clear cell carcinoma. (H & E stain, 20×).

in 50% of cases,[12] deletion of *PTEN* and a tumor suppressor gene involved in the *PI3K/PTEN* signaling pathway in 20%.[13] In addition to these results, single nucleotide polymorphism array analysis has established a deletion of the CDKN2A/2B locus and amplification of the ZNF2017 locus, which identify the important role of these pathways in the development of clear cell carcinoma of the ovary.[13]

Low-grade endometrioid carcinoma

The origin of low-grade endometrioid carcinoma resembles the origin of clear cell carcinoma. Both develop from endometriotic cysts and are associated with implants of endometriosis outside the ovaries.[11] Intrinsic genetic abnormalities were observed in eutopic endometrium found in patients with endometriosis.[14] The genetics and molecular pathogenesis of low-grade endometrioid carcinoma are similar to the pathogenesis of clear cell carcinoma. The mutations that affect the *PI3KCA/PTEN* signaling pathway are common in low-grade endometrioid carcinoma.[15] Deregulation of the Wnt/β-catenin signaling pathway was observed in 40% of endometrioid ovarian carcinomas. This pathway plays an important role in proliferation, motility, and survival. Abnormalities of the Wnt/β-catenin signaling pathway may rely on activation of mutation of *CTNNB1*, a gene that encodes β-catenin.[16] The mutation of *CTNNB1* has been associated with well-known features of low-grade endometrioid carcinoma such as squamous differentiation, low grade, and a relatively good prognosis.[17–19]

Mucinous carcinoma

Mucinous carcinomas are not well understood because they are rare (3% of epithelial ovarian cancers). Mucinous carcinomas (see **Fig. 1**B) have a strong association with *KRAS* mutations (75%). *KRAS* mutations have been shown in mucinous carcinomas and adjacent mucinous cystadenomas and borderline tumors supporting tumor progression in ovarian mucinous neoplasms.[20,21] Many studies have shown that most gastrointestinal-type tumors that involve the ovary are secondary.[22] The origin of mucinous tumors and Brenner tumors is challenging, because unlike serous, endometrioid, and clear cell tumors, they do not display a müllerian phenotype. Some researchers have suggested that mucinous tumors have a relationship to the endocervix; the mucinous epithelium that characterizes them more closely resembles gastrointestinal mucosa. The association of Brenner tumors and mucinous tumors has been well recognized. A study reported that after extensive sectioning, mucinous cystadenomas contained foci of Brenner tumor in 18% of cases.[23] Frequently, mucinous tumors were associated with Walthard cell nests, which are composed of benign transitional-type epithelium and are found frequently in paraovarian and paratubal locations. This similarity raises the possibility that mucinous tumors and Brenner tumors have the same origin.[24] Ovarian mature cystic teratomas have been suggested as an origin of gastrointestinal-type mucinous tumors.[25]

Type II Carcinomas

Serous carcinoma

Serous carcinoma represents about 70% of ovarian malignancies.[26] The epithelium of serous carcinomas is similar to fallopian tube epithelium, especially HGSCs (see **Fig. 1**A). These similarities suggest the fallopian origin of ovarian HGSC.[27] In the past, the fallopian tubes were not examined thoroughly because of a logical assumption that the precursors of ovarian carcinomas are in the ovaries and not in the fallopian tubes. However, in the last few years, this idea has changed dramatically and now many researchers believe that serous tubal intraepithelial carcinoma (STIC) may be the precursor of HGSC, especially if this lesion is in the fimbria.[8,20] Some studies show that STIC was found in 50% to 60% of patients who have negative *BRCA* mutations (ie, sporadic ovarian cancer).[28–32] A gene profiling study showed that the profile of gene expression in HGSC is more related to fallopian tube epithelium than the epithelium of the ovarian surface.[33] The identical *TP53* mutations in STIC and HGSC support the theory that STIC is a precursor of HGSC.[33–35] Further studies have confirmed that both HGSA and STIC share expression of *p53*, *p16*, *Rsf-1*, *FAS*, and *cyclin E1*.[35] HGSCs express *PAX8*, a müllerian marker, but do not express calretinin, a mesothelial marker that is seen in ovarian epithelium.[36] During ovulation, the fimbria of the fallopian tube come close to the ovary, which may explain the implantation of fallopian epithelium onto the surface of the ovary and cortical inclusion cyst formation. The free radical environment of ovulation itself and other factors such as inflammation may play a role in ovarian carcinogenesis.[36] This is consistent with epidemiologic studies that showed the risk of ovarian cancers decreases with anovulation (oral contraceptive, multiparty).[37,38]

High-grade endometrioid carcinomas

Although low-grade endometrioid carcinomas are easily recognized, it is difficult to distinguish between high-grade endometrioid carcinoma (see **Fig. 1**C) and HGSC. This similarity raises the question whether high-grade endometrioid carcinoma is a variant of HGSC. These difficulties reflect the genetics and molecular similarities between high-grade endometrioid carcinomas and HGSC. Low-grade endometrioid carcinomas have mutations that deregulate the canonical Wnt/β-catenin and *PI3K/PTEN* signaling pathways and lack *TP53* mutations, whereas high-grade endometrioid carcinomas lack Wnt/β catenin or *PI3K/PTEN* signaling pathway defects and frequently have *TP53* mutations.[17] A few high-grade endometrioid carcinomas exhibit mutations found in low-grade endometrioid carcinomas in addition to *TP53* mutations, which suggest that some low-grade endometrioid carcinomas may progress to high-grade carcinomas. Similar findings have been seen in serous tumors, so the general consensus is that low-grade and high-grade carcinomas develop independently but rarely does a low-grade tumor progress to a high-grade tumor. The high frequency of *TP53* mutation that occurs in both high-grade endometrioid carcinoma and HGSC suggests that they both develop in a similar fashion and explains why high-grade endometrioid carcinoma is closely related to HGSC.

Clinical Implications of the Dualistic Model of Ovarian Carcinogenesis

Molecular and genetics studies have led to better understanding of the pathogenesis of epithelial ovarian carcinomas. The old concepts regarding the origin of epithelial ovarian carcinoma as ovarian have been changed and these new concepts will have many clinical implications and will help in improving early detection and management of ovarian neoplasms.

Some researchers argue that type I tumors do not need urgent biomarker screening tests because they are slow growing, present as a large mass when diagnosed, and are still confined to the ovaries. They are easy to detect by pelvic ultrasonography or pelvic examination and responsible for about 10% of ovarian cancer deaths.[25] On the other hand, type II tumors constitute 75% of ovarian cancers, account for approximately 90% of ovarian cancer deaths,[25] and are rarely confined to the ovaries at diagnosis. These features of type II tumors emphasize the importance of developing a screening or biomarker test that detects very small tumors even if outside the ovary.

For type I tumors confined to the ovary, oophorectomy alone may be sufficient treatment in some cases. Chemotherapy is effective if these tumors spread outside the ovary. Understating of the pathogenesis and deregulation of signaling pathways may lead to new medications. For instance, mutations in *KRAS* or *BRAF* may cause activation of the MAPK signaling pathway, so it is logical to assume that MAPK kinase inhibitors could benefit survival.

In contrast, treatment of type II tumor should start early. Early treatment depends on the development of a new screen or biomarkers that detect the tumor at an early stage. Inactivation of the *BRCA1/BRCA2* pathway may induce death in cancer cells. This approach has been tested in preclinical and clinical ovarian cancers with poly (ADP-ribose) polymerase (PARP) inhibitors such as olaprid and AG0114699. It is likely that PARP inhibitors will be effective in treating type II tumors.[39,40]

UTERINE CARCINOMAS: MOLECULAR FEATURES AND PATHOGENESIS

Two types of endometrial carcinoma (EC) are distinguished with respect to biology and clinical course. Type I carcinoma is related to hyperestrogenism by association with endometrial hyperplasia, which usually develops in perimenopausal women with frequent expression of estrogen and progesterone receptors, whereas type II carcinoma is unrelated to estrogen, associated with atrophic endometrium, frequent lack of estrogen and progesterone receptors, and older age.[41]

By histology, endometrioid and mucinous carcinomas are considered type I, and serous and clear cell carcinomas are type II. Among these, the most frequent tumor type is endometrioid adenocarcinoma (**Fig. 2**B) and they can show many histologic variants including villoglandular pattern, secretory changes, and squamous differentiation.[41] It has also been shown that molecular alterations involved in the development of type I carcinomas are different from type II carcinoma.

Type I Uterine Carcinoma

Four main molecular genetic alterations have been described in type I uterine carcinoma: microsatellite instability (MSI), which occurs in 25% to 30% of cases; *PTEN*

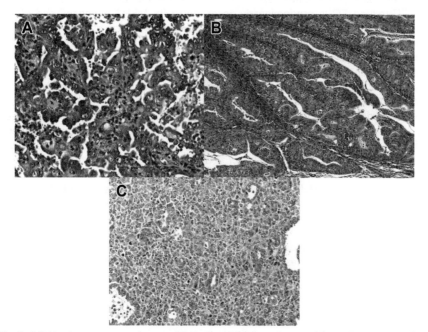

Fig. 2. (*A*) Uterine serous carcinoma. (*B*) Endometrioid carcinoma. (*C*) Carcinosarcoma. (H & E stain, 20×).

mutations in 37% to 61%; *kRAS* mutations in 10% to 30%; and CTNNB1 mutations with nuclear protein accumulation in 25% to 38% of cases. Although MI, *PTEN*, or *kRAS* mutations may coexist in many cases, these molecular abnormalities are not usually associated with β-catenin alterations. Type II tumors exhibit alterations of *p53*, loss of heterozygosity (LOH) on several chromosomes, as well as other molecular alterations (STK15, p16, E-cadherin, and C-erb B2).

MSI

Microsatellite DNA sequences are short tandem repeats distributed throughout the genome. The most common dinucleotide sequence in eukaryotes is the (CA)n repeat, and there are 50,000 to 100,000 (CA)n repeats in the entire human genome. The genes responsible for MI encode proteins involved in DNA mismatch repair (hMSH-2, hMLH-1, hPMS1, or hPMS2). Mutations of these genes alter the ability of the cells to repair errors produced during DNA replication. Therefore, cells with mutated mismatch repair genes replicate DNA mistakes more frequently than normal cells.[42]

MSI was initially found in cancers from patients with the hereditary nonpolyposis colon cancer (HNPCC) syndrome; it was also found in some sporadic tumors. EC is the second most common neoplasm encountered in patients with HNPCC. MSI has been detected in 75% of cases of EC associated with HNPCC but also in 25% to 30% of cases of sporadic EC.[42] Histopathologic features suggestive of HNPCC-related carcinoma are well characterized in the colon but not in the uterus. However, when examining an EC in a patient less than 50 years of age or with a personal or family history of colon carcinoma, it is important to consider the possibility of an HNPCC-related endometrial carcinoma. In these cases, testing for defective DNA mismatch repair may be performed by immunohistochemistry (MSH1, MLH2, MLH6, and PMS2 antibodies are commercially available). Loss of MSH2 expression essentially always indicates Lynch syndrome and MSH6 is related to MSH2. HNPCC-related EC is predominantly associated with MSH2 mutations and MLH6 mutations in particular. PMS2 loss is often associated with loss of MLH1 and is only independently meaningful if MLH1 is intact. In addition, polymerase chain reaction assays can be used to detect high levels of microsatellite alterations (MSI), a condition that is definitive for defective DNA mismatch repair. This testing is performed on paraffin-embedded tissue and compares the results of tumor DNA with those of non-neoplastic tissues from the same patient.

Although data are controversial regarding the prognostic significance of MI, it is usually associated with a high histologic grade. Patients who have HNPCC and EC have an inherited germ line mutation in MLH-1, MSH-2, MSH-6, or PMS-2 (first hit); but EC develops only after the instauration of a deletion or mutation in the contralateral MLH-1,MSH-2, MSH-6, or PMS-2 allele (second hit) in endometrial cells.[43–45] Once the 2 hits occur, the deficient mismatch repair role of the gene (MLH-1, MSH-2, MSH-6, or PMS-2) causes the acquisition of MSI, and the development of the tumor. In sporadic EC, MLH-1 inactivation by promoter hypermethylation is the main cause of mismatch repair deficiency, which usually occurs at the precursor (atypical hyperplasia) lesion. Thus, MLH-1 hypermethylation is an early event in the pathogenesis of type I carcinoma, which precedes the development of MSI. The prognostic significance of MI is under debate, but there is some convincing evidence suggesting an association with favorable outcome.[42–45]

PTEN

The tumor suppressor gene termed *PTEN*, located at chromosome10q23, encodes a protein (phosphatase and tensin homolog, PTEN) with tyrosine kinase function and behaves as a tumor suppressor gene. PTEN has been reported to be altered in up to 83% of endometrioid carcinomas and 55% of precancerous lesions. PTEN inactivation is caused by mutations that lead to a loss of expression and, to a lesser extent, by a LOH. Thus, loss or altered PTEN expression results in aberrant cell growth and apoptotic escape. Loss of PTEN is furthermore probably an early event in endometrial tumorigenesis, as shown by its presence in precancerous lesions, and is likely initiated in response to known hormonal risk factors. Its expression is highest in an estrogen-rich environment; in contrast, progesterone promotes involution of PTEN-mutated endometrial cells.

LOH at the PTEN region occurs in 40% of cases of EC. Somatic PTEN mutations are also common and found predominantly in Endometrioid Endometrial Carcinoma (EEC), occurring in 37% to 61% of cases. PTEN mutations have been identified in endometrial hyperplasias with and without atypia (19% and 21%, respectively).[46] Furthermore, PTEN mutations have been detected in hyperplasias coexisting with MI-positive EC, which suggests that PTEN mutations are early events in the development of EC. Data are controversial regarding the prognostic significance of PTEN mutations in EC, but there are some results that suggest an association with favorable prognostic factors.[47] This testing is performed on paraffin-embedded tissue, using immunohistochemistry.

The RAS-RAF-MEK-ERK signaling pathway

The RAS-RAF-MEK-ERK signaling pathway plays an important role in tumorigenesis. The frequency of kRAS mutations in EC ranges between 10% and 30%. In some series, KRAS mutations have been reported to be more frequent in EC showing MI. During tumorigenesis, activated RAS is usually associated with enhanced proliferation, transformation, and cell survival. BRAF, another member of the RAS-RAF-MEK-ERK pathways, is infrequently mutated in EC. RAS effectors like RASSF1A are supposed to have an inhibitory growth signal, which needs to be inactivated during tumorigenesis. RASSF1A inactivation by promoter hypermethylation may contribute significantly to increased activity of the RAS-RAF-MEK-ERK signaling pathway.[44]

PIK3CA

Mutations in PIK3CA, which codes for the p110α catalytic subunit of PI3K, have been described in various tumors and may contribute to the alteration of the PI3K/AKT signaling pathway in EC. PI3K is a heterodimer enzyme consisting of a catalytic subunit and a regulatory subunit.

The PIK3CA gene, located on chromosome3q26.32, codes for the p110a catalytic subunit of PI3K. A high frequency of mutations in the PIK3CA gene has been reported recently in EC. Mutations are located predominantly in the helical (exon 9) and kinase (exon 20) domains, but they can also occur in exons 1 to 7. PIK3CA mutations occur in 24% to 39% of cases, and coexist frequently with PTEN mutations. Oda and colleagues[48] described mutations in the PIK3CA gene in ECs for the first time. In this series, PIK3CA mutations occurred in 36% of cases, and coexisted frequently with PTEN mutations. Subsequent studies have shown that PIK3CA mutations, particularly in exon 20, are frequent in EC, and are associated with adverse prognostic factors such as high histologic grade, myometrial invasion, and vascular invasion.

β-Catenin gene (CTNNB1)

The β-catenin gene (CTNNB1) maps to 3p21. β-Catenin seems to be important in the functional activities of both APC and E-cadherin. β-Catenin is a component of the E-cadherin-catenin unit, which is important for cell differentiation and maintenance of the normal tissue architecture. β-Catenin is also important in signal transduction.[49] Mutations in exon 3 of *CTNNB1* result in stabilization of the β-catenin protein, cytoplasmic and nuclear accumulation, and participation in signal transduction and transcriptional activation through the formation of complexes with DNA binding proteins.[44,50] They seem to be independent of the presence of MI, and the mutational status of *PTEN* and *kRAS*. These mutations are believed to be homogeneously distributed in different areas of the tumors, which suggest that they do play a role in the early steps of endometrial tumorigenesis. Alterations in β-catenin have been described in endometrial hyperplasias that contain squamous metaplasia (morules). Data are controversial regarding the prognostic significance of β-catenin mutations in EC, but they probably occur in tumors with good prognosis.[51,52]

In routine practice, pathologists are faced with tumors showing mixed, morphologic, and molecular characteristics. Serous and clear cell carcinomas have been classified within the same category of type II carcinomas, based on high nuclear grade and aggressive behavior. However, recent studies have shown that these carcinomas are actually distinct tumor types.[44] They exhibit different clinical, immunohistochemical, and molecular features. Another controversial setting is cases between high-grade (predominantly solid) type I and type II ECs. Distinction between these 2 types of tumors is difficult; conversely, high-grade type I EC occasionally exhibits molecular alterations typical of type II EC such as *TP53* mutations. Because of the controversial prognostic usefulness and therapeutic modalities, MSI testing and PTEN are routinely offered using paraffin-embedded tissue, however the role of other molecular tests in daily practice has yet to be elucidated.

Treatment modalities
Recent advances in understanding of the molecular and genetic basis of EC have led to the development of targeted therapies that inhibit cellular signaling pathways involved in cell growth and proliferation. Several of these targeted agents are currently being investigated in EC. Inactivating mutations of *PTEN*, a tumor suppressor gene, are found in 40% to 60% of endometrial cancers. PTEN-deficient cells are sensitive to mammalian target of rapamycin (mTOR) inhibitors in vitro because loss of PTEN leads to constitutive activation of Akt, which in turn upregulates mTOR activity. Hence, there was interest in testing mTOR inhibitors in the treatment of EC. These inhibitors are expected to be effective in cancers like EC with *PTEN* mutations, *PIKECA* mutations, and receptor tyrosine kinase-dependent activation. Combinations of mTOR inhibitors with hormonal therapy, chemotherapy, or other targeted therapies such as epidermal growth factor receptor (EGFR) inhibitors and antiangiogenic agents have been promising in the preclinical setting, and numerous trials to develop and test such combinations are under way.

Type II Uterine Carcinoma

Type II uterine carcinomas arise in postmenopausal women, are associated with atrophy, and by definition are graded as high grade. These tumors are reported to have a poor prognosis.

These include:

1. Serous carcinoma
2. Clear cell carcinoma
3. Carcinosarcoma

Uterine serous carcinoma

Uterine serous carcinomas accounting for approximately 15% of cases, approximately 50% of deaths due to uterine carcinomas are caused by this subtype.[53] This highlights the aggressive nature of this disease compared with the more indolent endometrioid carcinoma and its variants. Significant differences in survival have been reported between stage-matched serous carcinoma and FIGO grade 3 endometrioid carcinoma; serous carcinomas have lower survival.[53] In most cases, the tumor presents at a late stage with extrauterine involvement possibly the underlying cause of the poor prognosis of these tumors.[54–56] The rate of recurrence even in seemingly limited disease is high ranging from 31% to 80%.[57–59] More recent data have shown that low-stage disease, confined to the endometrium and polyp, was associated with a poor outcome.[60] Even the presence of a small amount of serious histology (<10%) in an EC is reported to have a poorer prognosis compared with pure grade 3 endometrioid carcinoma.[61]

Histologically, the morphology of this tumor, as described by Hendrickson and colleagues,[62] is similar to ovarian serous carcinoma. Cytologically, high-grade nuclei with gland formation/clefting and papillary configuration with floating tufts of neoplastic cells make up the morphology of this tumor (see **Fig. 2**A). It is well documented that uterine serous carcinomas are more common in older women[63] and have been described in an atrophic background.[64] Increasing evidence shows that endometrial intraepithelial carcinoma (EIC) is the precursor of uterine serous carcinoma. This lesion is described as malignant cells lining the surface of the endometrium or glands without invasion.

TP53 The most common mutation seen in uterine serous carcinoma is mutations in the *p53* gene. This is a tumor suppressor gene present on chromosome 17p and its activities include cell cycle control and apoptosis. Loss of the normal activity prevents apoptosis and promotes tumor progression.[65] Mutations in this gene result in an abnormal protein, which although dysfunctional, is more stable and can be stained by immunohistochemistry.[66] Other mutations prevent transcription of any protein and thus show no staining by immunohistochemistry.[65] These alterations have been reported in about 90% of cases of serous carcinoma.[65] It has been postulated that the hypoxic environment of atrophic endometrium promotes selection of cells, which are able to overcome apoptosis, thereby selecting for cells that already contain *p53* mutations. In addition, these mutations have also been documented in EIC and concordant mutations occurring in the EIC component and concurrent serous carcinoma have also been identified, implying that these mutations occur early in the pathogenesis of serous carcinomas.[65]

Her-2/neu The success of trastuzumab in breast cancer treatment has led to interest in assessing this gene and its function in EC.

Her-2/neu receptor is a membrane-bound tyrosine kinase receptor with an extracellular ligand-binding domain, a transmembrane component, and an intracellular component related to tyrosine kinase enzyme. Her-2/neu gene amplification results in overexpression of the receptors with homodimerization and ultimately in activation of the tyrosine kinase enzyme and related pathways, resulting in increased cell proliferation.[67]

Variable levels of Her-2/neu protein expression and gene amplification have been reported in uterine serous carcinomas,[68] with a lack of concordance between the two. This most likely is due to the small number of cases in each study. Higher levels of Her-2/neu expression have been reported in African Americans with this disease alluding to race-related biological differences affecting this tumor type.[68] A relatively poor prognosis has been attributed to tumors bearing overexpression and amplification of Her-2/neu, including recurrence and overall survival.[69,70] Although it has prognostic significance, treatment with trastuzumab does not seem to confer any benefit to these patients.

EGFR EGFR is a transmembrane tyrosine kinase receptor (belonging to the same family as Her-2), similarly composed of an extracellular ligand-binding domain, intracellular tyrosine kinase activity, and a portion spanning the cell membrane. Ligands associated with EGFR are EGF and transforming growth factor α. Mutant variants of EGFR, although they do not bind a ligand, have activated tyrosine kinase resulting in increased cell progression and inhibition of apoptosis. Although the studies are limited in the literature, EGFR overexpression has been reported in a significant subset of serous carcinomas although *EGFR* mutations were not documented in these cases.[71,72] However, downstream *PIK3CA* mutations were identified in a small proportion of these cases.[72] The purpose of identifying these mutations in addition to understanding the pathogenesis of these tumors provides a foundation for new therapeutic molecules.

Other alterations seen more frequently in serous carcinomas are p16 inactivation and decreased E-cadherin expression.[73] Mutation analyses have identified a high frequency of mutations involving *TP53* as expected, *PPP2R1A*, and *PI3KCA*.[74]

Clear cell carcinoma

These tumors have a distinctive histologic appearance composed of cuboidal cells with clear or eosinophilic cytoplasm, hyalinized cores, extracellular globules, and hyperchromatic nuclei. The cells exhibit hob nailing and are arranged in glandular and papillary configurations (see **Fig. 2**B). They are often present in association with serous carcinoma as mixed tumors. They are associated with a poor prognosis.

Meaningful studies on this tumor type have been limited because of its rarity. Although some degree of *p53* alterations are seen in clear cell carcinoma, they seems to be much less compared with serous carcinoma. Also, *PTEN* mutations are rare and reported *KRAS* mutations are rare.[75] EGFR is reported to be overexpressed.[76]

Carcinosarcoma (malignant mixed müllerian tumor)

These tumors comprise 2% to 5% of all ECs. Although more commonly reported in the postmenopausal age group, they have been reported in younger women who might have undergone pelvic radiation for unrelated causes.[77] Stage for stage, this subtype has a poorer prognosis than other subtypes.[78]

Morphologically, these tumors are composed of carcinomatous and sarcomatous components, which are intimately admixed with each other (see **Fig. 2**C). Studies have concluded that the 2 components are clonal. Recent studies have shown immunohistochemical expression of p53, MSH2, and MSH6 corresponding to epithelial and mesenchymal components, confirming the monoclonal origin of uterine carcinosarcomas. Therefore, the proposal that these tumors represent metaplasia of the carcinomatous component into sarcomatous components is being increasingly accepted.[77,79] Chromosomal alterations were identified using comparative genomic hybridization analysis. Gains were seen more commonly than losses (85% vs 30%). The epithelial component is either endometrioid or serous, whereas the sarcomatous component is composed of homologous or heterologous elements. Mutational analyses have subtyped carcinosarcomas into 2 categories: the serous type with *TP53* and *PPP2R1A* mutations and the endometrioid type with mutations involving *PTEN* and *ARID1A*.[74] As expected, p53 expression is associated with a nonendometrioid epithelial tumor component and expression patterns of MMR proteins, PTEN, and hormone receptors are seen in endometrioid component carcinomas.[80]

SUMMARY

Understanding the molecular basis of EC helps to provide an explanation for the prognosis of these tumors. Also, this understanding opens up avenues for research into novel therapies that may prove beneficial.

REFERENCES

1. Boyle P, Levin B. World cancer report 2008. Lyon (France): World Health Organization; 2008.
2. Siegel R, Naishadham D, Jemal A. Cancer statistics, 2013. CA Cancer J Clin 2013;63(1):11–30.
3. Shih Ie M, Kurman RJ. Ovarian tumorigenesis: a proposed model based on morphological and molecular genetic analysis. Am J Pathol 2004;164(5): 1511–8.
4. Jones S, Wang TL, Shih Ie M, et al. Frequent mutations of chromatin remodeling gene ARID1A in ovarian clear cell carcinoma. Science 2010;330(6001): 228–31.
5. Ahmed AA, Etemadmoghadam D, Temple J, et al. Driver mutations in TP53 are ubiquitous in high grade serous carcinoma of the ovary. J Pathol 2010;221(1): 49–56.
6. Karamurzin Y, Leitao MM Jr, Soslow RA. Clinicopathologic analysis of low-stage sporadic ovarian carcinomas: a reappraisal. Am J Surg Pathol 2013;37(3): 356–67.
7. Plaxe SC. Epidemiology of low-grade serous ovarian cancer. Am J Obstet Gynecol 2008;198(4):459.e1–8 [discussion: 459.e8–9].
8. Vang R, Shih Ie M, Kurman RJ. Fallopian tube precursors of ovarian low- and high-grade serous neoplasms. Histopathology 2013;62(1):44–58.
9. Prat J. New insights into ovarian cancer pathology. Ann Oncol 2012;23(Suppl 10):x111–7.
10. Yamamoto S, Tsuda H, Takano M, et al. Clear-cell adenofibroma can be a clonal precursor for clear-cell adenocarcinoma of the ovary: a possible alternative ovarian clear-cell carcinogenic pathway. J Pathol 2008;216(1):103–10.
11. Veras E, Mao TL, Ayhan A, et al. Cystic and adenofibromatous clear cell carcinomas of the ovary: distinctive tumors that differ in their pathogenesis and behavior: a clinicopathologic analysis of 122 cases. Am J Surg Pathol 2009; 33(6):844–53.
12. Campbell IG, Russell SE, Choong DY, et al. Mutation of the PIK3CA gene in ovarian and breast cancer. Cancer Res 2004;64(21):7678–81.
13. Sato N, Tsunoda H, Nishida M, et al. Loss of heterozygosity on 10q23.3 and mutation of the tumor suppressor gene PTEN in benign endometrial cyst of the ovary: possible sequence progression from benign endometrial cyst to endometrioid carcinoma and clear cell carcinoma of the ovary. Cancer Res 2000;60(24): 7052–6.
14. Bulun SE. Endometriosis. N Engl J Med 2009;360(3):268–79.
15. Obata K, Morland SJ, Watson RH, et al. Frequent PTEN/MMAC mutations in endometrioid but not serous or mucinous epithelial ovarian tumors. Cancer Res 1998;58(10):2095–7.

16. Cho KR, Shih Ie M. Ovarian cancer. Annu Rev Pathol 2009;4:287–313.

17. Wu R, Hendrix-Lucas N, Kuick R, et al. Mouse model of human ovarian endometrioid adenocarcinoma based on somatic defects in the Wnt/beta-catenin and PI3K/Pten signaling pathways. Cancer Cell 2007;11(4):321–33.

18. Gamallo C, Palacios J, Moreno G, et al. Beta-catenin expression pattern in stage I and II ovarian carcinomas: relationship with beta-catenin gene mutations, clinicopathological features, and clinical outcome. Am J Pathol 1999;155(2): 527–36.

19. Saegusa M, Okayasu I. Frequent nuclear beta-catenin accumulation and associated mutations in endometrioid-type endometrial and ovarian carcinomas with squamous differentiation. J Pathol 2001;194(1):59–67.

20. Kurman RJ, Shih Ie M. Molecular pathogenesis and extraovarian origin of epithelial ovarian cancer–shifting the paradigm. Hum Pathol 2011;42(7): 918–31.

21. Gemignani ML, Schlaerth AC, Bogomolniy F, et al. Role of KRAS and BRAF gene mutations in mucinous ovarian carcinoma. Gynecol Oncol 2003;90(2): 378–81.

22. Riopel MA, Ronnett BM, Kurman RJ. Evaluation of diagnostic criteria and behavior of ovarian intestinal-type mucinous tumors: atypical proliferative (borderline) tumors and intraepithelial, microinvasive, invasive, and metastatic carcinomas. Am J Surg Pathol 1999;23(6):617–35.

23. Seidman JD, Khedmati F. Exploring the histogenesis of ovarian mucinous and transitional cell (Brenner) neoplasms and their relationship with Walthard cell nests: a study of 120 tumors. Arch Pathol Lab Med 2008;132(11):1753–60.

24. Seidman JD, Yemelyanova A, Zaino RJ, et al. The fallopian tube-peritoneal junction: a potential site of carcinogenesis. Int J Gynecol Pathol 2011;30(1):4–11.

25. Vang R, Gown AM, Zhao C, et al. Ovarian mucinous tumors associated with mature cystic teratomas: morphologic and immunohistochemical analysis identifies a subset of potential teratomatous origin that shares features of lower gastrointestinal tract mucinous tumors more commonly encountered as secondary tumors in the ovary. Am J Surg Pathol 2007;31(6):854–69.

26. McCluggage WG. Morphological subtypes of ovarian carcinoma: a review with emphasis on new developments and pathogenesis. Pathology 2011;43(5): 420–32.

27. Erickson BK, Conner MG, Landen CN Jr. The role of the Fallopian tube in the origin of ovarian cancer. Am J Obstet Gynecol 2013. http://dx.doi.org/10.1016/j.ajog.2013.04.019.

28. Callahan MJ, Crum CP, Medeiros F, et al. Primary fallopian tube malignancies in BRCA-positive women undergoing surgery for ovarian cancer risk reduction. J Clin Oncol 2007;25(25):3985–90.

29. Shaw PA, Rouzbahman M, Pizer ES, et al. Candidate serous cancer precursors in fallopian tube epithelium of BRCA1/2 mutation carriers. Mod Pathol 2009; 22(9):1133–8.

30. Finch A, Shaw P, Rosen B, et al. Clinical and pathologic findings of prophylactic salpingo-oophorectomies in 159 BRCA1 and BRCA2 carriers. Gynecol Oncol 2006;100(1):58–64.

31. Medeiros F, Muto MG, Lee Y, et al. The tubal fimbria is a preferred site for early adenocarcinoma in women with familial ovarian cancer syndrome. Am J Surg Pathol 2006;30(2):230–6.

32. Przybycin CG, Kurman RJ, Ronnett BM, et al. Are all pelvic (nonuterine) serous carcinomas of tubal origin? Am J Surg Pathol 2010;34(10):1407–16.

33. Marquez RT, Baggerly KA, Patterson AP, et al. Patterns of gene expression in different histotypes of epithelial ovarian cancer correlate with those in normal fallopian tube, endometrium, and colon. Clin Cancer Res 2005;11(17):6116–26.
34. Lee Y, Miron A, Drapkin R, et al. A candidate precursor to serous carcinoma that originates in the distal fallopian tube. J Pathol 2007;211(1):26–35.
35. Sehdev AS, Kurman RJ, Kuhn E, et al. Serous tubal intraepithelial carcinoma up-regulates markers associated with high-grade serous carcinomas including Rsf-1 (HBXAP), cyclin E and fatty acid synthase. Mod Pathol 2010;23(6):844–55.
36. Kurman RJ, Shih Ie M. The origin and pathogenesis of epithelial ovarian cancer: a proposed unifying theory. Am J Surg Pathol 2010;34(3):433–43.
37. Beral V, Bull D, Green J, Reeves G, Million Women Study Collaborators. Ovarian cancer and hormone replacement therapy in the Million Women Study. Lancet 2007;369(9574):1703–10.
38. Lurie G, Thompson P, McDuffie KE, et al. Association of estrogen and progestin potency of oral contraceptives with ovarian carcinoma risk. Obstet Gynecol 2007;109(3):597–607.
39. Audeh MW, Carmichael J, Penson RT, et al. Oral poly(ADP-ribose) polymerase inhibitor olaparib in patients with BRCA1 or BRCA2 mutations and recurrent ovarian cancer: a proof-of-concept trial. Lancet 2010;376(9737):245–51.
40. Tutt A, Robson M, Garber JE, et al. Oral poly(ADP-ribose) polymerase inhibitor olaparib in patients with BRCA1 or BRCA2 mutations and advanced breast cancer: a proof-of-concept trial. Lancet 2010;376(9737):235–44.
41. Llobet D, Pallares J, Yeramian A, et al. Molecular pathology of endometrial carcinoma; practical aspects from the diagnostic and therapeutical view points. J Clin Pathol 2009;62:777–85.
42. Caduff RF, Johnston CM, Svoboda-Newman SM, et al. Clinical and pathological significance of microsatellite instability in sporadic endometrial carcinoma. Am J Pathol 1996;148:1671–8.
43. Duggan BD, Felix JC, Muderspach LI, et al. Microsatellite instability in sporadic endometrial carcinoma. J Natl Cancer Inst 1994;86:1216–21.
44. Matias-Guiu X, Prat J. Molecular pathology of endometrial carcinoma. Histopathology 2013;62(1):111–23.
45. Kobayashi K, Sagae S, Kudo R, et al. Microsatellite instability in endometrial carcinomas: frequent replication errors in tumors of early onset and/or of poorly differentiated type. Genes Chromosomes Cancer 1995;14:128–32.
46. Risinger JI, Berchuck A, Kohler MF, et al. Genetic instability of microsatellites in endometrial carcinoma. Cancer Res 1993;53:5100–3.
47. Matias-Guiu X, Catasus L, Bussaglia E, et al. Molecular pathology of endometrial hyperplasia and carcinoma. Hum Pathol 2001;32:569–77.
48. Oda K, Stokoe D, Taketani Y, et al. High frequency of coexistent mutations of PIK3CA and PTEN genes in endometrial carcinoma. Cancer Res 2005;65:10669–73.
49. Catasus L, Matias-Guiu X, Machin P, et al. Frameshift mutations at coding mononucleotide repeat microsatellites in endometrial carcinomas with microsatellite instability. Cancer 2000;88:2290–7.
50. Catasus L, Gallardo A, Cuatrecasas M, et al. PIK3CA mutations in the kinase domain (exon 20) of uterine endometrial adenocarcinomas are associated with adverse prognostic parameters. Mod Pathol 2008;21:131–9.
51. Catasus L, D'Angelo E, Pons C, et al. Expression profiling of 22 genes involved in the PI3K–AKT pathway identifies two subgroups of high-grade endometrial carcinomas with different molecular alterations. Mod Pathol 2010;23:694–702.

52. Rudd ML, Price JC, Fogoros S, et al. A unique spectrum of somatic PIK3CA (p110alpha) mutations within primary endometrial carcinomas. Clin Cancer Res 2011;17:1331–40.

53. Slomovitz BM, Burke TW, Eifel PJ, et al. Uterine papillary serous carcinoma (UPSC): a single institution review of 129 cases. Gynecol Oncol 2003;91:463–9.

54. Trope C, Kristensen GB, Abeler VM. Clear-cell and papillary serous cancer: treatment options. Best Pract Res Clin Obstet Gynaecol 2001;15:433–46.

55. Matthews RP, Hutchinson-Colas J, Maiman M, et al. Papillary serous and clear cell type lead to poor prognosis of endometrial carcinoma in black women. Gynecol Oncol 1997;65:206–12.

56. Soslow RA, Bissonnette JP, Wilton A, et al. Clinicopathologic analysis of 187 high-grade endometrial carcinomas of different histologic subtypes: similar outcomes belie distinctive biologic differences. Am J Surg Pathol 2007;31: 979–87.

57. Wu W, Slomovitz BM, Celestino J, et al. Coordinate expression of Cdc25B and ER-alpha is frequent in low-grade endometrioid endometrial carcinoma but uncommon in high-grade endometrioid and nonendometrioid carcinomas. Cancer Res 2003;63:6195–9.

58. Naumann RW. Uterine papillary serous carcinoma: state of the state. Curr Oncol Rep 2008;10:505–11.

59. Bristow RE, Asrari F, Trimble EL, et al. Extended surgical staging for uterine papillary serous carcinoma: survival outcome of locoregional (Stage I-III) disease. Gynecol Oncol 2001;81:279–86.

60. Semaan A, Mert I, Munkarah AR, et al. Clinical and pathologic characteristics of serous carcinoma confined to the endometrium: a multi-institutional study. Int J Gynecol Pathol 2013;32:181–7.

61. Boruta DM 2nd, Gehrig PA, Groben PA, et al. Uterine serous and grade 3 endometrioid carcinomas: is there a survival difference? Cancer 2004;101:2214–21.

62. Hendrickson M, Ross J, Eifel P, et al. Uterine papillary serous carcinoma: a highly malignant form of endometrial adenocarcinoma. Am J Surg Pathol 1982;6:93–108.

63. Lachance JA, Everett EN, Greer B, et al. The effect of age on clinical/pathologic features, surgical morbidity, and outcome in patients with endometrial cancer. Gynecol Oncol 2006;101:470–5.

64. Ambros RA, Sherman ME, Zahn CM, et al. Endometrial intraepithelial carcinoma: a distinctive lesion specifically associated with tumors displaying serous differentiation. Hum Pathol 1995;26:1260–7.

65. Tashiro H, Isacson C, Levine R, et al. p53 gene mutations are common in uterine serous carcinoma and occur early in their pathogenesis. Am J Pathol 1997;150: 177–85.

66. Reihsaus E, Kohler M, Kraiss S, et al. Regulation of the level of the oncoprotein p53 in non-transformed and transformed cells. Oncogene 1990;5:137–45.

67. Perez-Soler R. HER1/EGFR targeting: refining the strategy. Oncologist 2004;9: 58–67.

68. Santin AD, Bellone S, Van Stedum S, et al. Amplification of c-erbB2 oncogene: a major prognostic indicator in uterine serous papillary carcinoma. Cancer 2005; 104:1391–7.

69. Slomovitz BM, Broaddus RR, Burke TW, et al. Her-2/neu overexpression and amplification in uterine papillary serous carcinoma. J Clin Oncol 2004;22: 3126–32.

70. Lukes AS, Kohler MF, Pieper CF, et al. Multivariable analysis of DNA ploidy, p53, and HER-2/neu as prognostic factors in endometrial cancer. Cancer 1994;73: 2380–5.

71. Konecny GE, Venkatesan N, Yang G, et al. Activity of lapatinib a novel HER2 and EGFR dual kinase inhibitor in human endometrial cancer cells. Br J Cancer 2008;98:1076–84.

72. Hayes MP, Douglas W, Ellenson LH. Molecular alterations of EGFR and PIK3CA in uterine serous carcinoma. Gynecol Oncol 2009;113:370–3.

73. Holcomb K, Delatorre R, Pedemonte B, et al. E-cadherin expression in endometrioid, papillary serous, and clear cell carcinoma of the endometrium. Obstet Gynecol 2002;100:1290–5.

74. McConechy MK, Ding J, Cheang MC, et al. Use of mutation profiles to refine the classification of endometrial carcinomas. J Pathol 2012;228:20–30.

75. Lax SF. Molecular genetic pathways in various types of endometrial carcinoma: from a phenotypical to a molecular-based classification. Virchows Arch 2004; 444:213–23.

76. Khalifa MA, Mannel RS, Haraway SD, et al. Expression of EGFR, HER-2/neu, P53, and PCNA in endometrioid, serous papillary, and clear cell endometrial adenocarcinomas. Gynecol Oncol 1994;53:84–92.

77. Yamada SD, Burger RA, Brewster WR, et al. Pathologic variables and adjuvant therapy as predictors of recurrence and survival for patients with surgically evaluated carcinosarcoma of the uterus. Cancer 2000;88:2782–6.

78. Amant F. The rationale for comprehensive surgical staging in endometrial carcinosarcoma. Gynecol Oncol 2005;99:521–2 [author reply: 522–3].

79. McCluggage WG. Uterine carcinosarcomas (malignant mixed Mullerian tumors) are metaplastic carcinomas. Int J Gynecol Cancer 2002;12:687–90.

80. de Jong RA, Nijman HW, Wijbrandi TF, et al. Molecular markers and clinical behavior of uterine carcinosarcomas: focus on the epithelial tumor component. Mod Pathol 2011;24:1368–79.

Index

Note: Page numbers of article titles are in **boldface** type.

A

Abbott Molecular Assay, for melanocytic neoplasms, 883–884
Abelson murine leukemia virus oncogene homolog 1, 828
ABO blood group, 809–810
AccuProbe assays, 788–789
Acute leukemia with mixed lineage leukemia translocation, 825–826
Acute lymphoblastic leukemia, 825–826
Acute myeloid leukemia, 824–827, 831
Acute promyelocytic leukemia, 824
Adenoid cystic carcinoma, of breast, 902
Adenoma-carcinoma sequence, in colorectal carcinoma, 836–838
Affirm VPIII microbial identification test, 791–792
Alloimmune thrombocytopenia, platelet antigens in, 814
All-trans retinoic acid, for hematopoietic malignancies, 831
AML 1 protein, in leukemia, 825
Ampullary adenocarcinoma, 862
Amsterdam criteria, for colorectal carcinoma, 839
Anaplastic lymphoma kinase translocation assay, for lymphomas, 823–824
Androgen receptors, in breast carcinoma, 896, 900–901
Angiopoietins, in hepatic adenomas, 877
AntagomiRs, 778
Antibodies, in transfusion medicine, **805–816**
Antigens, in transfusion medicine, **805–816**
APC gene pathway
    in colorectal cancer, 837–839, 852
    in small intestinal adenocarcinoma, 863
Apocrine carcinoma, of breast carcinoma, 896, 900
Appendix, adenocarcinoma of, **861–866**
ARID1 gene
    in ovarian cancer, 912
    in uterine carcinoma, 920
Array comparative genomic hybridization, for melanocytic neoplasms, 885
ATRA, for leukemia, 831

B

B cells, clonal populations of, 818–820
Basal-like subtype, of breast carcinoma, 895–896
B-cell leukemia/lymphoma-2 (BCL-2) translocation assay, for lymphomas, 820–821
BCL-2 gene, in breast carcinoma, 899
BCL-2 like protein 11, 822
BCL-2 translocation assay, for lymphomas, 820–821

Clin Lab Med 33 (2013) 927–939
http://dx.doi.org/10.1016/S0272-2712(13)00085-1
0272-2712/13/$ – see front matter © 2013 Elsevier Inc. All rights reserved.

labmed.theclinics.com

United States Postal Service

Statement of Ownership, Management, and Circulation
(All Periodicals Publications Except Requestor Publications)

1. Publication Title	2. Publication Number	3. Filing Date
Clinics in Laboratory Medicine	0 0 0 - 7 1 1 3	9/14/13

4. Issue Frequency	5. Number of Issues Published Annually	6. Annual Subscription Price
Mar, Jun, Sep, Dec	4	$240.00

7. Complete Mailing Address of Known Office of Publication *(Not printer) (Street, city, county, state, and ZIP+4®)*

Elsevier Inc.
360 Park Avenue South
New York, NY 10010-1710

Contact Person
Stephen R. Bushing

Telephone *(Include area code)*
215-239-3688

8. Complete Mailing Address of Headquarters or General Business Office of Publisher *(Not printer)*

Elsevier Inc., 360 Park Avenue South, New York, NY 10010-1710

9. Full Names and Complete Mailing Addresses of Publisher, Editor, and Managing Editor *(Do not leave blank)*

Publisher *(Name and complete mailing address)*

Linda Belfus, Elsevier, Inc., 1600 John F. Kennedy Blvd. Suite 1800, Philadelphia, PA 19103-2899

Editor *(Name and complete mailing address)*

Patrick Manley, Elsevier, Inc., 1600 John F. Kennedy Blvd. Suite 1800, Philadelphia, PA 19103-2899

Managing Editor *(Name and complete mailing address)*

Barbara Cohen - Kligerman, Elsevier, Inc., 1600 John F. Kennedy Blvd. Suite 1800, Philadelphia, PA 19103-2899

10. Owner *(Do not leave blank. If the publication is owned by a corporation, give the name and address of the corporation immediately followed by the names and addresses of all stockholders owning or holding 1 percent or more of the total amount of stock. If not owned by a corporation, give the names and addresses of the individual owners. If owned by a partnership or other unincorporated firm, give its name and address as well as those of each individual owner. If the publication is published by a nonprofit organization, give its name and address.)*

Full Name	Complete Mailing Address
Wholly owned subsidiary of	1600 John F. Kennedy Blvd., Ste. 1800
Reed/Elsevier, US holdings	Philadelphia, PA 19103-2899

11. Known Bondholders, Mortgagees, and Other Security Holders Owning or Holding 1 Percent or More of Total Amount of Bonds, Mortgages, or Other Securities. If none, check box ☐ None

Full Name	Complete Mailing Address
N/A	

12. Tax Status *(For completion by nonprofit organizations authorized to mail at nonprofit rates) (Check one)*
The purpose, function, and nonprofit status of this organization and the exempt status for federal income tax purposes:
☐ Has Not Changed During Preceding 12 Months
☐ Has Changed During Preceding 12 Months *(Publisher must submit explanation of change with this statement)*

PS Form 3526, September 2007 (Page 1 of 3 (Instructions Page 3)) PSN 7530-01-000-9931 PRIVACY NOTICE: See our Privacy policy in www.usps.com

---

13. Publication Title	14. Issue Date for Circulation Data Below
Clinics in Laboratory Medicine	September 2013

15. Extent and Nature of Circulation			Average No. Copies Each Issue During Preceding 12 Months	No. Copies of Single Issue Published Nearest to Filing Date
a. Total Number of Copies *(Net press run)*			330	337
b. Paid Circulation (By Mail and Outside the Mail)	(1)	Mailed Outside-County Paid Subscriptions Stated on PS Form 3541. *(Include paid distribution above nominal rate, advertiser's proof copies, and exchange copies)*	139	137
	(2)	Mailed In-County Paid Subscriptions Stated on PS Form 3541 *(Include paid distribution above nominal rate, advertiser's proof copies, and exchange copies)*		
	(3)	Paid Distribution Outside the Mails Including Sales Through Dealers and Carriers, Street Vendors, Counter Sales, and Other Paid Distribution Outside USPS®	52	68
	(4)	Paid Distribution by Other Classes Mailed Through the USPS (e.g. First-Class Mail®)		
c. Total Paid Distribution *(Sum of 15b (1), (2), (3), and (4))*		▶	191	205
d. Free or Nominal Rate Distribution (By Mail and Outside the Mail)	(1)	Free or Nominal Rate Outside-County Copies Included on PS Form 3541	56	57
	(2)	Free or Nominal Rate In-County Copies Included on PS Form 3541		
	(3)	Free or Nominal Rate Copies Mailed at Other Classes Through the USPS (e.g. First-Class Mail)		
	(4)	Free or Nominal Rate Distribution Outside the Mail (Carriers or other means)		
e. Total Free or Nominal Rate Distribution *(Sum of 15d (1), (2), (3) and (4))*		▶	56	57
f. Total Distribution *(Sum of 15c and 15e)*		▶	247	262
g. Copies not Distributed *(See instructions to publishers #4 (page #3))*		▶	83	75
h. Total *(Sum of 15f and g)*		▶	330	337
i. Percent Paid (15c divided by 15f times 100)			77.33%	78.24%

16. Publication of Statement of Ownership

☐ If the publication is a general publication, publication of this statement is required. Will be printed in the December 2013 issue of this publication. ☐ Publication not required

17. Signature and Title of Editor, Publisher, Business Manager, or Owner

(signature) Stephen R. Bushing – Inventory Distribution Coordinator

Date September 14, 2013

I certify that all information furnished on this form is true and complete. I understand that anyone who furnishes false or misleading information on this form or who omits material or information requested on the form may be subject to criminal sanctions (including fines and imprisonment) and/or civil sanctions (including civil penalties).

PS Form 3526, September 2007 (Page 2 of 3)

Printed and bound by CPI Group (UK) Ltd, Croydon, CR0 4YY

03/10/2024

01040478-0020